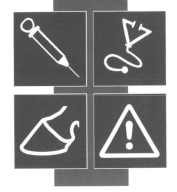

YOUR Horse's Health
FIRST AID

ANNA RUSH

MRCVS

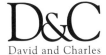

D&C
David and Charles

Anna was born into a Suffolk farming family, educated at Framlingham College and then Bristol University, from where she graduated with a degree in Veterinary Science in 2000. Since graduating she has worked in mixed practice in the UK and Australia. Anna is married with one spaniel, and harbours a desire to ski every day.

A DAVID & CHARLES BOOK
Copyright © David & Charles Limited 2008

David & Charles is an F+W Publications Inc. company
4700 East Galbraith Road
Cincinnati, OH 45236

First published in the UK in 2008

Text copyright © Anna Rush 2008
Photographs copyright © Anna Rush 2008 except those listed below

Pages 18, 19, 20, 22, 26, 39 (right, middle and lower left), 40 (lower left and middle), 44 (left), 45 (lower right), 48, 50 (right), 53, 55, 58, 61, 65, 66, 68, 70 (left), 76, 80 (lower), 86, 88 (lower), 89 (top), 90, 97 (right), 100 (top left), 105 (top left), 106 (top left and right), 107, 110 (lower), 112 (left), 113 (top), 114 (lower right and left), 115, 120 (top), 112–3, 128, 134, 135, 136, 140 (top), 141 and 150 copyright © Karen Coumbe 2008

Pages 4–5,36–7,41 (top right), 43, 63 (top), 69 (third row right and second from right), 72 (top right), 77 (lower), 81, 84, 87 (lower left), 89 (lower), 91 (lower left), 93 (lower right), 98 (top and middle), 104, 105 (top right), 109 (top), 110 (top), 111 (left), 114 (top), 126, 129, 131, 132,133,138–9, 144 (top), 146, 148 and 149 copyright © Horsepix 2008. With its roots in horse country and staffed by horse people, Horsepix is a leading provider of high quality equestrian photography.

Page 108 by Matthew Roberts copyright © David & Charles Limited 2008

Page 111 (right) copyright © Frank Ruedisueli 2008

Page 124 copyright © PunchStock/ThinkStock 2008

Page 125 copyright © AFP/Getty Images 2008

Page 147 copyright © Sue Devereux 2008

Illustrations by Maggie Raynor copyright © David & Charles Limited 2008 except those on page 43 by Visual Image, 78 and 92 by Ethan Danielson and 92 and 93 by Jodie Lystor copyright © David & Charles Limited 2008

A catalogue record for this book is available from the British Library.

ISBN-13: 978-0-7153-2773-9 hardback
ISBN-10: 0-7153-2773-9 hardback

Printed in China by RR Donnelley
for David & Charles
Brunel House, Newton Abbot, Devon

Commissioning Editor: Jane Trollope
Editorial Manager: Emily Pitcher
Assistant Editor: Emily Rae
Project Editor: Anne Plume
Designers: Alistair Barnes and Jodie Lystor
Production Controller: Beverley Richardson

Visit our website at www.davidandcharles.co.uk

David & Charles books are available from all good bookshops; alternatively you can contact our Orderline on 0870 9908222 or write to us at FREEPOST EX2 110, D&C Direct, Newton Abbot, TQ12 4ZZ (no stamp required UK only); US customers call 800-289-0963 and Canadian customers call 800-840-5220.

Contents

3

INTRODUCTION

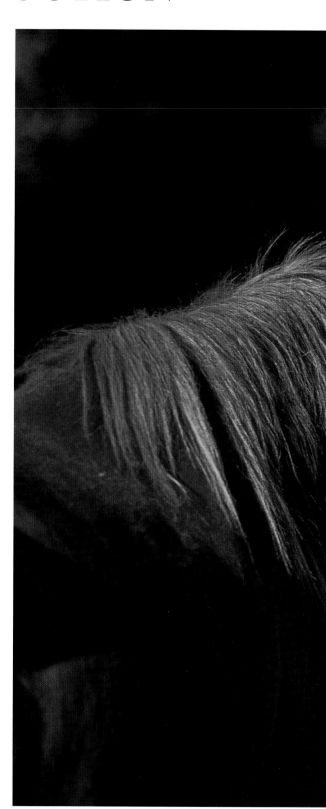

Owning a horse is a huge responsibility, and at times quite stressful. *Your Horse's Health: First Aid* explains how to tell if your horse is healthy, and what to do if you think something is wrong. It clearly sets out how to take control of a situation and minimize the damage, giving you the confidence to treat simple problems yourself. Problems that have the potential to be very serious are highlighted so that you can recognize them and take appropriate action rapidly.

This simple, logical approach to the horse and first aid situations is divided into four main sections:

Section 1 General first aid. Covers wound care and bandaging and general medical know-how. This section explains what is normal and healthy and what is not; and how to perform basic first aid care and what equipment you should have to help you cope with most situations.

Section 2 Overview of the body systems. Works through the horse's body systematically by organ system. Each system section includes what symptoms to look for and their relative seriousness, what to do to minimize the problem, when you can deal with it yourself and when you should call the vet, as well as an explanation of how the vet is likely to treat the problem. Never forget that your vet is on the end of the phone for advice, and that a vet is available 24 hours a day.

Section 3 How to approach emergency situations. Gives an outline of the important things to consider in a range of emergency situations such as a road traffic accident or getting stuck in a ditch; these are when it is most important to have a clear head, but when you are most likely to be given a wide range of different advice – so having a clear plan in your head is really important to help you stay calm if the worst should happen.

Section 4 Diagnostic procedures and treatment. Provides an explanation of diagnostic procedures and treatments that might be used by your vet, to help you understand what your vet is doing and why.

A glossary and explanation of the technical veterinary words used in the text will help to demystify treatments and improve communication between you and your vet.

Finally, building a positive relationship with your vet is one of the best things you can do for you and your horse!

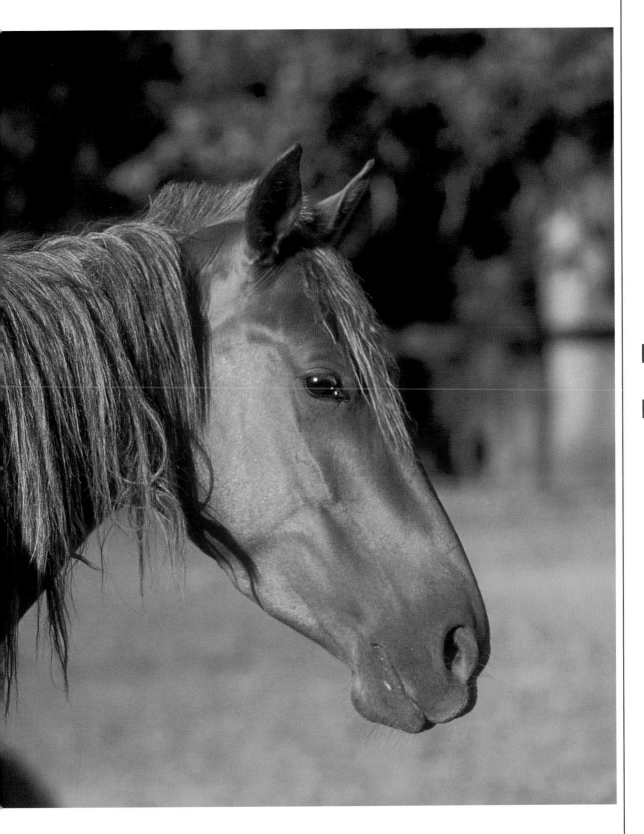

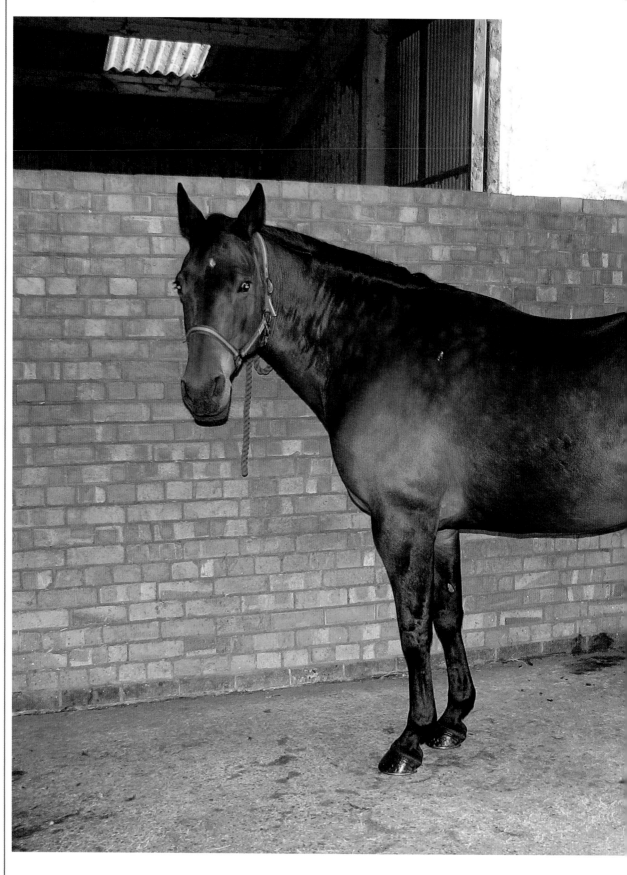

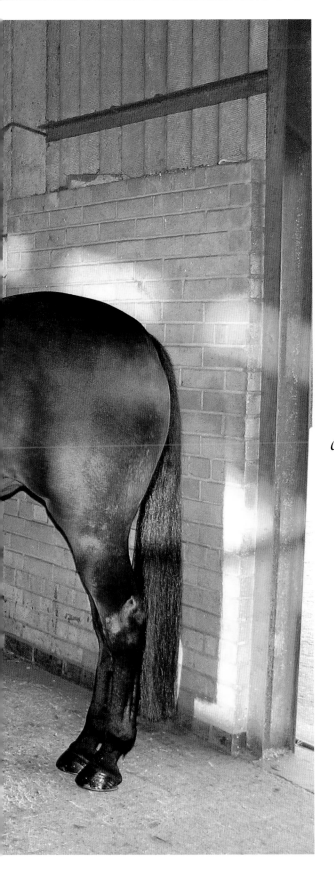

SECTION 1
GENERAL
FIRST AID

This section covers general first aid, explaining how to monitor the basic health parameters of your horse, and enabling you to recognize when a problem is developing. Bandaging and wound dressing techniques are clearly explained and illustrated.

7

MONITORING BASIC HEALTH PARAMETERS

FIRST AID FACTS

Knowing your horse in its normal healthy state is very important in its daily care: if you know what is normal you will be able to recognize quickly when something is wrong.

A horse's appearance, or its basic health parameters – for example its temperature and pulse – will alter if there is a medical problem. Measuring body temperature and taking a pulse are quantifiable ways to measure the health of your horse, and any alterations in the circulation will also give you an indication of your horse's health.

You should check your horse over for wounds at least twice a day, for instance when he comes out of the stable and when he comes in from the field.

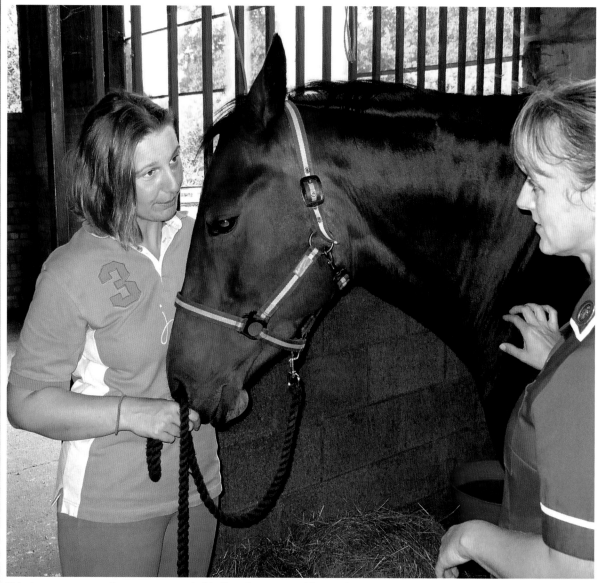

Veterinary nurses can be more approachable than the vet, providing an important link between you and your practice

TAKING A TEMPERATURE

Check your thermometer is working correctly: mercury thermometers need to be shaken down so that the mercury level is as close to the neck of the bulb as possible; digital thermometers need to be turned on, and the display checked. Apply lubrication, such as Vaseline or KY jelly, to the end of the thermometer.

For your own safety, ask another person to steady the head of your horse, then proceed as follows:

- Approach your horse down the near side as though you were going to pick up a hind foot.
- When you reach the back leg, stand close to your horse, use your left hand to move the tail sideways, and with your right hand gently insert the thermometer into the anus. Hold the thermometer at an angle so that you can feel its end lying against the rectal wall.
- Leave the thermometer in place for 1 minute (mercury) or until it beeps (digital), then remove it carefully, and read it.
- A normal temperature is between 100.8 and 102.5°F/ 37.4 and 39.0°C.

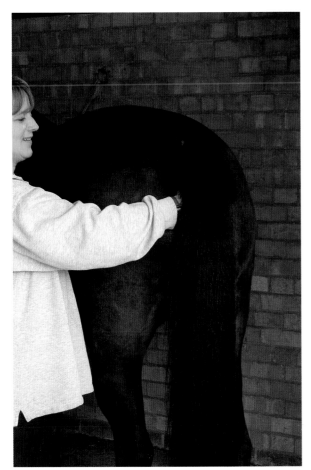

Standing to one side of the horse is an important safety precaution when taking the temperature

TAKING A PULSE

Monitoring the pulse gives a good measure of health, including fitness and pain levels. It's much easier to find the pulse on a Thoroughbred, so if you can, try checking on finer-coated horses to start with. Once you are confident that you know where to locate it, then you can progress to thicker-skinned, thicker-coated horses such as cobs.

The pulse rate will increase with exercise, excitement, pain and raised temperature. Normal pulse rates vary between individuals, but should be between 25–40 beats per minute. It can be quite difficult to feel the pulse in a fit, healthy horse as it is so slow, so practise on your horse immediately after exercise when the pulse should be raised.

Some very fit horses occasionally drop a beat at rest; if this happens while you are monitoring the pulse you will feel a random double space between heartbeats, and then the pulse continuing at a steady pace. The first time you come across this it can be quite alarming!

Feeling the pulse on the jawline
Feel along the bottom edge of the cheek until you find a bundle of vessels about halfway along. Gently apply pressure with your fingers until you can feel the pulse.

Feeling the heartbeat
If your horse is a bit fidgety or you are struggling to feel the pulse along the jawline, then you can feel the heart directly. Place the flat of your hand on your horse's chest wall about one hand's width behind the elbow; you should feel the heart beating. This is the same position that is used to listen for the heart with a stethoscope.

Feeling the pulse on the fetlock
Put your thumb on one side and your first two fingers on the opposite side of the fetlock at the base of the cannon bone. Gradually slide your fingers and thumb backwards across the fetlock until you feel a bundle of vessels on either side. Gradually increase the pressure with your fingers until you can feel the pulse.

This is a very useful pulse to be able to feel to monitor inflammation in the foot, for instance abscesses or laminitis: the strength of the pulse will increase noticeably with increasing inflammation.

Feeling the pulse on the pastern

Using your first two fingers, start at the middle of the pastern at the back of the leg, and gradually move your fingers towards the outside until you feel a bundle of vessels.

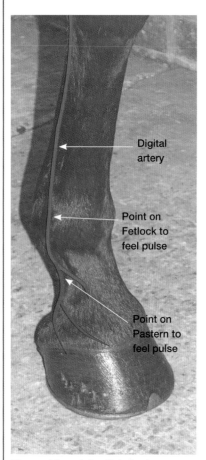

Digital artery

Point on Fetlock to feel pulse

Point on Pastern to feel pulse

Cartoid artery

Facial artery

Site to feel pulse

The position of the digital pulses

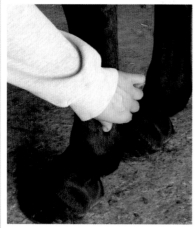

The fetlock pulse is easiest to find at the widest part of the joint

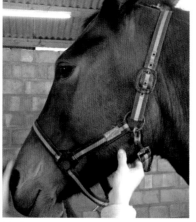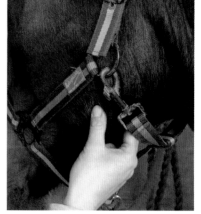

Feel carefully along the bottom of the cheek for the pulse by running your fingers along the inside of the cheekbone until you feel a bundle of vessels

SIGNS OF A HEALTHY CIRCULATION

- Deep salmon pink colour of the gums and the mucous membranes around the eyes.
- If pressure is applied to the gums the colour returns after a couple of seconds.
- If the skin is picked up between the fingers it returns to its normal position quickly.
- The pulse is strong and regular.
- Breathing is quiet and calm at rest.
- No build-up of fluid around the body, especially under the abdomen.

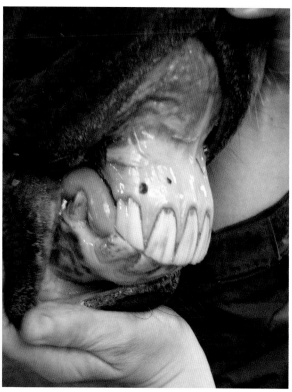

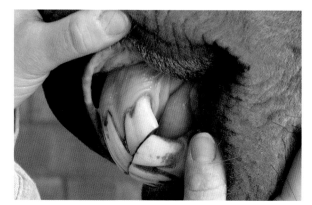

This illustrates the variation in colour of the gums of healthy horses, and this is why it is important to know your own horse

MONITORING BREATHING

A normal horse takes between six and twenty breaths per minute when standing quietly in the stable. To monitor the respiration rate, stand quietly and watch for the chest wall moving in and out. You should not easily see your horse breathe at rest (unless it sighs), nor should the nostrils be flared.

TOP TIP

Any wheezing, squeaking, snoring or snorting at rest is abnormal, and it should be investigated. If you can see your horse making two movements to breathe out, one from the chest and one from the abdomen, this is a clear indicator of inflamed airways, often as a result of allergies.

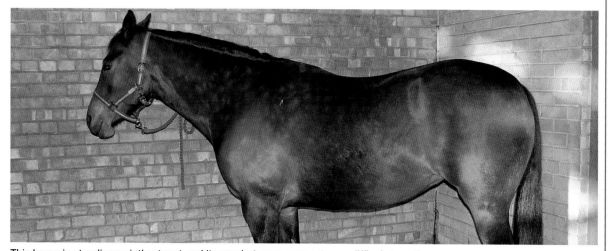

This horse is standing quietly at rest and its respiratory movements are difficult to notice

THE FIRST AID KIT

BARE FACTS

Your first aid kit needs to be kept in a dry, water-tight container in a place where it can be found quickly and easily (but not by mice). The following are useful contact numbers that should be kept with or in the first aid kit:

- vet clinic – plus mobile number if you have one
- farrier
- emergency contact for riders
- equine transport

EQUIPMENT

- Clean bucket or bowl.

- **Antiseptic**: either an iodine solution or antiseptic solution from the vet. This could be Savlon™, Hibiscrub™, Pevodine™ or an equivalent off-the-shelf anti-bacterial cleaner.

- **Gauze swabs**: are better for cleaning wounds than cotton wool, as fewer fibres are left in the wound.

- **Cotton wool**: can be used for padding in bandages, or for cleaning wounds if no swabs are available.

- **Gloves**: single-use latex gloves, or the equivalent if you have a sensitivity to latex. These will also protect the

wound from further contamination, and will protect you and your hands if the wound is infected.

- **Thermometer**: these can be either digital or mercury. Digital thermometers are easier to read; if you have a mercury thermometer make sure it is always shaken down before use.

- **Scissors**: blunt-ended, curved scissors if possible, but any will do as long as you are careful.

- **Antibiotic spray**: often referred to as 'blue spray', this is an aerosol containing Oxytetracycline, an antibiotic used to disinfect shallow wounds and grazes.

- **Petroleum jelly**: used mainly to soften scabs, but also useful to protect the skin from wounds which continue to weep for a prolonged period of time; for example, Vaseline™.

- **Torch**: put the batteries in back to front, then there is no risk of them draining and not working when you really need them.

- **Homoeopathic remedies**: for example, Rescue™ Remedy, arnica or any other products whose use is advised by an experienced or qualified homoeopath.

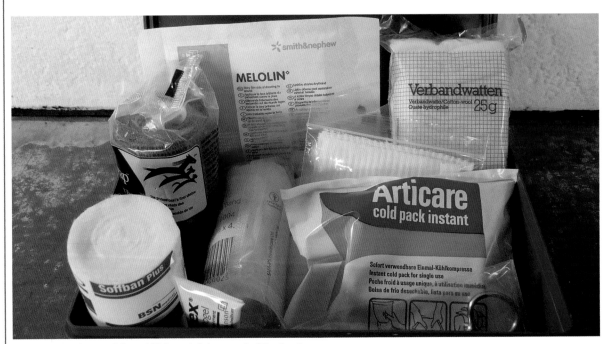

An example of a small first aid kit containing most of the basics

BANDAGES AND DRESSINGS

- **Wound dressing**: use a non-adhesive, sterile dressing such as Melonin™. Other dressings, such as charcoal-activated or **hydrophilic** dressings are available, but are designed for wounds that should be treated under veterinary supervision.

- **Wound gel** (hydrogel): is used to help keep deep wounds moist, and to draw debris and infective agents out, for example Intrasite™.

- **Poultice**: for foot abscesses – a square of plastic-backed, soft wadding such as the proprietary Animalintex™ or Poultex™.

- **Padding bandages**: rolls of cotton wool-like bandage used to pad between dressings and the outer layer of bandage, for example Soffban™ or Orthoban™.

- **Self-adhesive bandages**: are available in different widths; depending on where the bandage is to be applied, these bandages are stretchy and so conform to the contours of the horse's limb, for example Coform™ or Vetrap™.

- **Adhesive bandages**: help to prevent bandages slipping, for example Elastoplast™.

- **Hard-wearing sticky tape**: is used in place of boots to protect the bottom of poultices and foot bandages, for example Ducktape™.

- **Gamgee™ and stable bandages**: if there is any prolonged lameness then the opposite limb must have supportive bandaging in order to prevent strain or damage to the tendons in that leg from excessive weight-bearing.

- **Cooling bandages**: are used for tendon strains, but must be used with care to prevent cold injury to the skin and underlying tissues.

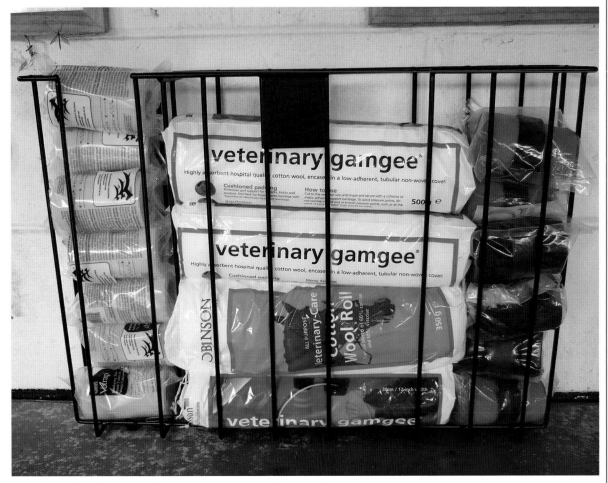

Keep a selection of clean bandages and dressings easily accessible

DEALING WITH WOUNDS

WOUND BASICS

A wound can be a graze, where the full thickness of the skin is not broken; a cut or laceration where the skin is broken and the tissues beneath are exposed; or a puncture, which is generally a deep injury with a small entry point – for example, where a sharp, slender, long **foreign body** has entered the flesh.

The depth, position and size of a wound will decide how serious an injury it is, and this will dictate the type of treatment required.

Tetanus infection is normally contracted from soil contamination of a wound, especially a deep puncture wound. It is important to make sure that your horse's tetanus vaccine is up to date at all times.

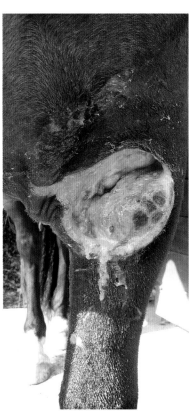
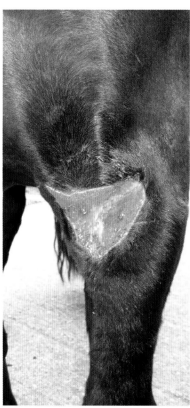
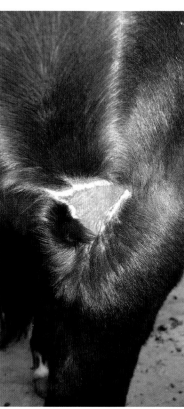

This extensive, contaminated wound was caused by a fall over a fence. It healed with careful management over a period of 3–4 months

---

HOW DOES A WOUND HEAL?

When a wound first occurs a blood clot fills the wound and the white blood cells in the blood clot start to clean up any debris or infection. As the clot matures it contracts and pulls the edges of the wound closer, and skin (epithelial) cells grow from the edge of the wound towards the centre.

Extensive wounds produce **granulation tissue** over four to five days, and this forms a bed for the epithelial cells to grow on while providing a strong defence against infection as a result of the very effective local immune system. Depending on the size of the wound, the epithelial cells will eventually cover the wound completely, forming a weak skin that eventually matures into normal skin or scar tissue, depending on how much tension it is under.

Wound contraction is the gradual movement of the surrounding skin inwards to shrink the wound and so reduce the area that requires new epithelial cells; this is most effective on areas of loose skin, such as the flanks. This contraction stops when either the skin becomes tight or **proud flesh** (see below, page 21) obstructs it.

GRAZES

FIRST AID FACTS
A graze is where the horse's coat has been rubbed off, but the full thickness of the skin is not broken. The depth, position and dimensions of a wound will decide how serious this sort of injury is, and this in turn will dictate the type of treatment that is required.

WHAT TO LOOK FOR
You should check your horse over for wounds at least twice a day – for instance, when he comes out of the stable to be turned out or ridden, and later, when he returns/ comes in from the field.

WHAT TO DO
- Grazes respond well to a thorough wash with an antiseptic solution, followed by being left alone.
- Topical treatments such as antibiotic aerosol ('blue spray') or wound powder can help protect the wound, but are not always necessary.
- Creams, on the other hand, often slow down healing and attract dirt to the wound.

WHAT YOUR VET MAY DO
It is unlikely that you will need the vet for a graze; however, if you are worried, do not hesitate to call them. Small grazes are usually treated with antiseptic solutions and – in some cases, depending on the cause of the injury – antibiotics.

Extensive grazes may require oral antibiotics, because the potential for infection is proportionately increased with a larger area of damage.

WHAT CAN GO WRONG
In some cases a bacterial infection can enter the body through the graze: this can cause either localized inflammation, or a more severe reaction called **cellulitis**.

Localized inflammation and infection can usually be controlled by improved wound care, but may require antibiotics if the infection is well established.

Cellulitis
Cellulitis is most commonly seen following a leg wound: usually an apparently insignificant wound appears to be healing when the leg suddenly swells dramatically. This rapid swelling is an over-reaction by the body to bacterial invaders.

To treat cellulitis usually requires antibiotics and anti-inflammatories, as well as regular cold hosing to reduce the swelling and bring the infection under control.

Severe cases of cellulitis can cause the skin to ooze fluid (**serum**); this fluid can scald the skin and cause a form of chemical burn. This is unusual and requires veterinary treatment immediately.

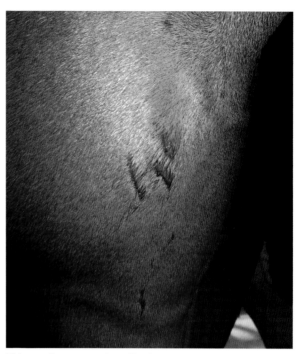

This small graze on the stifle does not require veterinary treatment

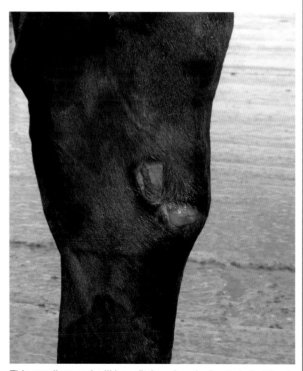

This small wound will benefit from bandaging to help it heal; as it is positioned over the hock, veterinary advice should be sought

CUTS AND LACERATIONS

FIRST AID FACTS

Cuts and/or lacerations are injuries that break the skin and expose the underlying tissues. The depth, position and size of this sort of wound will decide how serious it is, and this will dictate the level of treatment that is required to be given.

Tetanus is a bacterial infection normally contracted from soil contamination of a wound, especially a deep wound; it produces a toxin that causes all the muscles in the body to become stiff and inflexible, and can be fatal if not recognized and treated early – so ensure your horse's tetanus vaccine is up to date.

WHAT TO LOOK FOR

You should check your horse over for wounds at least twice a day – for instance, when he comes out of the stable or in from the field in the morning, and as the last thing you do before you leave him in the evening.

If a horse has sustained an injury in the field he may begin to act out of character, usually either being unwilling to be caught because he is in pain and frightened, or waiting by the gate for you to come and 'rescue' him.

WHAT TO DO

Small cuts and lacerations that are less than 3cm (1in) long and which go through the skin and not into underlying tissue will usually heal on their own.

Treatment of a small laceration should be as follows:

- Wash the cut with an antiseptic solution.
- Dry the area.
- Spray the wound with an antiseptic spray, or cover it with an antiseptic cream.
- Use a hydrogel if you suspect that there may still be debris in the wound.

- Only cover the wound if you feel that the cut will be damaged further without bandaging. (See Bandaging, page 22, for further information.)
- Check the wound again later in the day and continue to treat it as you would a wound on your own body.
- If the wound is bigger than 3cm (1in) long, or if you are worried, then call your vet for advice as it may need sutures or staples.

If you think the wound may need sutures, or the area around the wound is beginning to swell up, a simple dressing will help to minimize the swelling. This will also help to keep the cut edges of the skin together and will speed up healing.

> **TOP TIP**
>
> A thick coat can hide wounds, but usually any bleeding will result in the hair surrounding the injury becoming matted, and this can make the wound easier to find.

WHAT YOUR VET MAY DO

If you call the vet, remember to tell them when your horse was last vaccinated for tetanus.

Depending on the cause of the injury, the vet may give your horse pain relief, antibiotics to fight infection and antiseptics to clean the wound. They may also give you a lesson on the best way to bandage and treat your horse's wound in order to help it to heal as efficiently as possible.

If the vet feels the wound needs further investigation – for instance there is a foreign body or a complicated laceration – they may sedate the horse and use a local

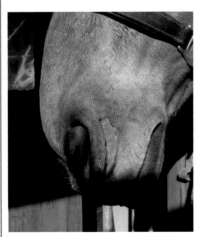
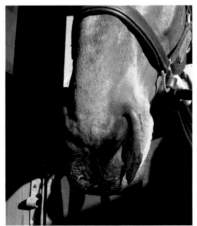
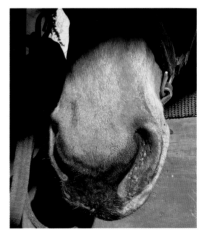

This extensive wound to the nostril was caused by the horse catching its head in the lorry. Following delicate suturing the entire flap was replaced into position, and it healed without complication and with a good cosmetic result

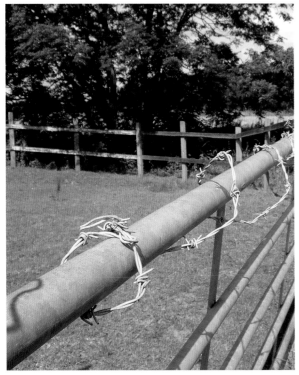
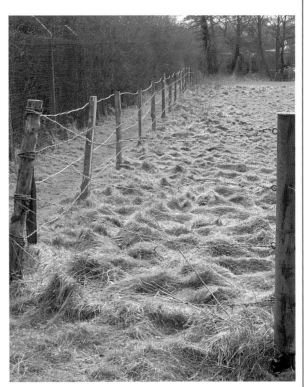

Barbed wire should not be used for fencing around horses. Loose fencing wire such as in the picture on the right is a greater risk for entanglement and laceration

anaesthetic in order to examine the injury. General anaesthesia will only be suggested in serious cases.

If the wound needs help in closing up, sutures or staples will be used. In this case sedation and local anaesthesia will usually be used to keep the horse calm during the treatment.

Lacerations will heal eventually, and often with little scarring, so don't panic if your horse cuts itself badly.

WHAT CAN GO WRONG

Deep lacerations can cause significant damage to underlying structures such as tendons and joints, depending on the location of the wound. Such wounds require urgent veterinary intervention.

Deep lacerations which include muscle can cause severe pain, and significant pain on movement; often physiotherapy is required to achieve full function of the limb after the initial recovery and healing.

Wound breakdown following suturing is common in areas where the skin normally moves a great deal (for example, over joints and the legs) or if there is excessive swelling or infection present. All wounds will heal eventually, but some may leave superficial scarring which can be unsightly.

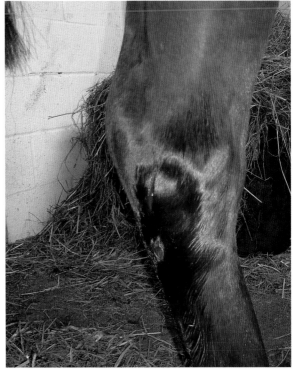

Although this is only a small wound, its location over the vulnerable hock joint means that it should be checked by a vet to make sure it is only superficial and does not involve the joint capsule

PUNCTURE WOUNDS

FIRST AID FACTS

A puncture wound is a deep injury with a small entry point, for example where a **foreign body** has entered the flesh. Foreign bodies can range in size from small thorns to steel nails or even bits of fence or hedge.

A wound's depth and size, and where it occurs on the horse's body, will decide how serious it is, and the type of treatment will be given accordingly.

Tetanus infections are normally contracted from soil contamination of a wound, and puncture wounds are the greatest risk, so you should always be sure that your horse's tetanus vaccine is up to date.

WHAT TO LOOK FOR

Most puncture wounds are to the foot, and are often the result of shoeing problems, such as a nail from a loose shoe or an old nail from a previous shoe.

WHAT TO DO

- Puncture wounds should be closely examined for depth and position.
- If the injury is in the foot or leg and the horse is not standing on it, call the vet.
- If you suspect the puncture wound is near a joint, call the vet immediately.
- If the injury is anywhere else on the body and you are at all concerned, call the vet.
- Bandaging and poulticing a puncture wound in the foot is covered in Bandaging and Poulticing, page 24.

WHAT YOUR VET MAY DO

When you call the vet, tell them when your horse was last vaccinated for tetanus.

Depending on the cause of the injury, the vet may give your horse pain relief, antibiotics to fight infection, antiseptics to clean the wound, and a lesson on the best way to bandage and treat the wound in order to help it heal as efficiently as possible.

If the vet feels the wound needs further investigation – for example, to explore the tract made by the foreign body, or to check if a joint or tendon sheath has been penetrated – they may sedate the horse and use a local anaesthetic to examine the injury. General anaesthesia will only be suggested in serious cases that require complete immobilization.

If a joint or a tendon sheath has been penetrated, then this is a very serious injury and requires flushing with sterile saline and aggressive antibiotic treatment. This may be done immediately, or your horse may be referred to a more specialized hospital or clinic for this more advanced treatment.

In some cases if the foreign body has broken off or fragmented, then a surgical exploration and cleaning of the wound may be required to remove any debris which

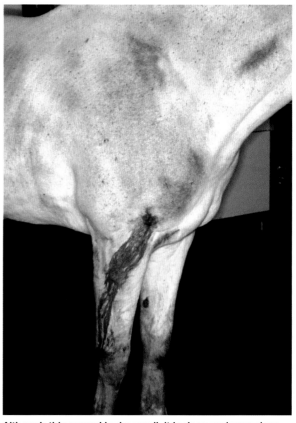

Although this wound looks small, it is deep and very close to the shoulder joint and will therefore require careful cleaning and investigation

> **TOP TIP**
>
> **If there is a foreign body in the horse's flesh, follow this advice:**
> - Leave the foreign body in place and call your vet for advice, as removing large foreign bodies can tear blood vessels and cause serious bleeding.
> - If the foreign body is sticking out from the horse's body *either* keep the horse somewhere where it cannot rub it or break it off, *or* place a supportive bandage around it so that it cannot be moved or knocked.

may harbour infection and slow down healing.

Usually puncture wounds do not require sutures as the external wound is small.

Puncture wounds to the feet are usually treated by aggressive flushing and poulticing (*see* page 24), sometimes in conjunction with **prophylactic antibiotics**.

WHAT CAN GO WRONG

Tetanus thrives in an **anaerobic** environment such as is produced by a deep, narrow puncture wound, so it is very important to ensure that every horse's tetanus vaccination is up to date.

Puncture wounds to the foot, if not noticed at the time, can develop into pus in the foot. This is a very painful condition which can normally be treated by paring the foot to release the pus; this should be done by either your farrier or your vet. In some cases the pus may track upwards and break through the coronary band. Once pus has been released, a poultice can then be used to draw out any that is remaining.

Puncture wounds that introduce infection into a joint or a tendon sheath can cause **septic arthritis**: this causes severe pain and must be treated aggressively, usually at a referral hospital as the initial flush is usually carried out under general anaesthesia. This condition cannot always be successfully treated, and can ultimately result in the euthanasia of the horse on welfare grounds.

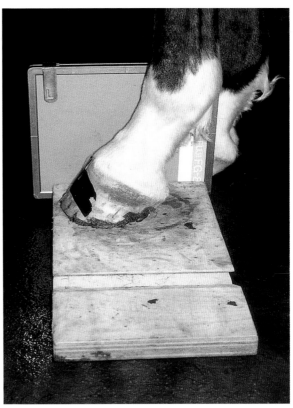

Puncture wounds to the foot may require an X-ray to check the damage

TOP TIP

Other bacterial infections, apart from tetanus, can develop in deep wounds, so they should be carefully monitored for inflammation and discharge.

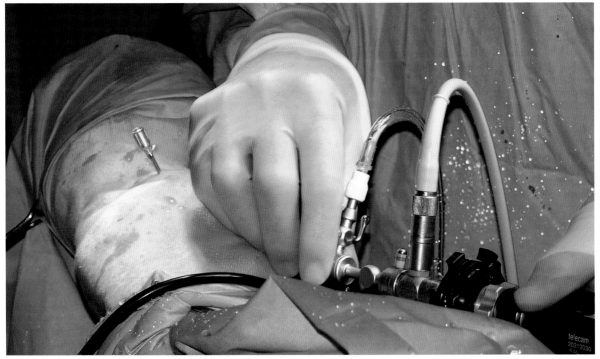

A rigid endoscope can be inserted directly into the joint to visualize the damage to the internal aspects of a joint as a result of a puncture wound. This must be performed under general anaesthetic with very strict aseptic precautions

BATHING A WOUND

WHAT YOU WILL NEED

- A bucket and a sponge or a hosepipe
- Plenty of clean, fresh water
- Antiseptic solution
- A jug or a clean bucket
- Swabs or cotton wool
- A clean towel to pat dry the area around the wound
- Correct dressing and bandage if required

HOW TO DO IT

- First wipe the area around the wound to remove superficial dirt that may contaminate the wound further, then move on to the wound itself, starting at the top and working your way down. A bucket and a sponge, or a hosepipe if your horse will tolerate it, work well for this, using plenty of clean, fresh water (with nothing in it); cold water will also help to slow the bleeding and ease the pain, albeit temporarily.
- Once the worst of the dirt has been removed, mix a small amount of antiseptic solution with some water in a jug or clean bucket.

- Then using gauze swabs (preferable to cotton wool as these do not leave fibres behind in the wound), clean the wound gently but thoroughly. Doing this will give you a better idea of how bad the wound actually is – many wounds look a lot better once the blood and mud has been washed away.
- Use a clean towel to pat as dry as possible the area all around the wound.
- If the wound requires a bandage you can apply the correct dressing now (see Bandaging, page 22).
- If you have a leg wound that you think will require suturing, apply a bandage once the wound is clean in order to minimize the swelling: this makes closing the wound an easier task for the vet, and reduces the risk of wound breakdown.

WHAT ELSE DO YOU NEED TO KNOW?

Most wounds heal quickly, on their own, with little intervention; even large wounds will heal eventually, often with minimal scarring. Not all wounds, even large ones, benefit from sutures – in some cases the sutures can hold infection in the wound and slow down the healing process.

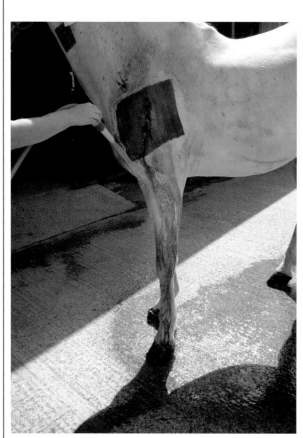

Cold hosing helps to decontaminate a wound and ease the discomfort

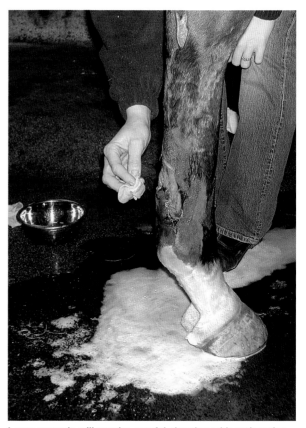

Large wounds will require careful cleaning with antiseptics before suturing can be attempted

WOUND BREAKDOWN

Wound breakdown is most commonly caused by contamination or infection interfering with the growth of new cells. The next most common problem is too much movement between the skin edges – this is why leg wounds tend to heal badly as the skin is tight and the movement of the leg keeps moving the skin edges away from each other. Some larger wounds that involve skin flaps, especially three-corner tears, may have problems healing because the blood supply to part of the flap has been damaged; this means that not enough nutrients are delivered to the wound, so the affected skin dies off, leaving a larger wound to heal.

Proud flesh is an overgrowth of **granulation** tissue, which is the early part of the healing process; it is most likely to occur if the wound is slow healing or if there is a large gap between the skin edges. Proud flesh does not have a nerve supply, so treatment is usually straightforward. The technique varies between vets, but generally relies on either the use of a **caustic** or a **steroid cream**, or cutting it off using a scalpel blade; this may need to be repeated, depending on the amount of proud flesh present. This should only be performed by your vet.

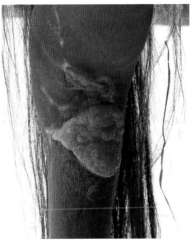

This large wound was caused by fencing wire becoming caught around the hock

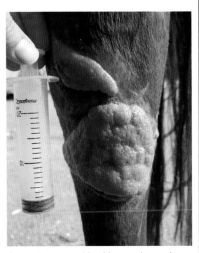

Once the wound had been cleaned and infection controlled, extensive proud flesh developed

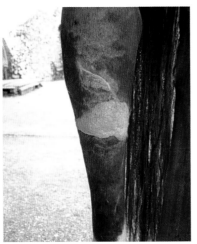

Removal of the proud flesh allowed the skin edges to start the healing process

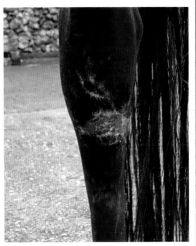

The wound one week on from the previous picture; with control of the proud flesh, healing is rapid. After two more weeks, healing was complete

BANDAGING

BANDAGING BASICS

There are a few basics that all horse owners should know about bandaging, so familiarize yourself, or refresh your memory, with the following:

- A bandage should always be clean and dry, with no odour or discharge striking through; if it is not, it should be removed immediately and the underlying limb/injury checked carefully.
- Always put on slightly more padding than you think will be necessary.
- The pressure of the bandage should be firm without being tight; serious damage can be done to the skin and underlying tissues if a tight bandage is left on for more than an hour.
- Self-adhesive bandages such as Vetrap™ or Coform™ are quite elasticated and must not be put on tightly; these bandages can also shrink if they become wet. Even pressure can be achieved by overlapping each turn of the bandage by approximately half the width of the bandage.
- If the bandage has slipped it should be removed immediately as it may be rubbing on the underlying limb/wound and exacerbating the primary injury.
- The edges of bandages should be checked regularly to ensure that straw, hay or shavings have not worked their way up under the bandage.

HOW DOES BANDAGING HELP WOUND HEALING?

Bandages help by protecting the wound from further contamination, reducing swelling, absorbing discharge, immobilizing the skin edges, and keeping the wound warm and moist. Care must be taken in the choice of dressing used next to the wound, because if the dressing sticks to the wound it will pull the new epithelial cells off when it is removed.

'Old Wives' Tales'

'MYTH':
It is not necessary to bandage a wound, just let the fresh air and sunshine heal it.

VET'S REPLY:
Any wound will heal eventually even if it is left alone without treatment, but the longer it takes to heal, the greater the risk of extensive scarring and long-term effects on the athletic ability of the horse. Without treatment and protection there is a much higher risk of infection, which can eventually affect the whole horse. Bandages help speed up the healing process significantly by producing the best conditions for healing; this means that the wound is kept warm and moist (but not wet), which encourages the growth of new tissue, and when a leg is bandaged correctly the dressing decreases the amount the leg can move and so helps keep the edges of the wound together.

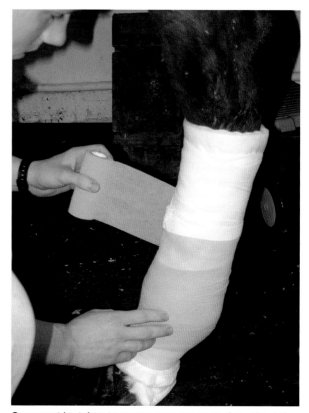

Care must be taken to ensure even pressure throughout the bandage to prevent slipping and rubbing

STABLE BANDAGES

'Stable bandages' are also known as 'support bandages'.

FIRST AID FACTS
Stable bandages are used when your horse is spending longer in the stable than he would usually. In particular, if your horse is lame on one leg it is important to ensure that a supportive bandage is put on the opposite leg in order to prevent subsequent strain or injury to that leg.

WHAT YOU WILL NEED
- Gamgee™ or protective material cut to fit your horse's leg: this needs to be long enough to cover the leg from above the knee to the hoof.
- Wide, slightly elasticated bandage.

HOW TO DO IT
Wrap the gamgee or protective under layer around the leg so that it reaches from just above the knee or hock to the coronet band; make sure the join is on the side of the leg away from the tendons.
- Starting on the canon near the knee, wrap the bandage from front to back.
- Gently but firmly wrap the stable bandage down the leg to just below the fetlock, then back up to just below the knee.
- Try to finish the bandage near the top or bottom of the canon bone.

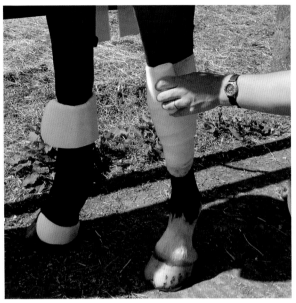

It is important to use a stable bandage on the opposite leg to an injury to prevent strain on the tendons if lameness is prolonged following the injury

WHAT ELSE DO YOU NEED TO KNOW?
Stable bandages should be checked and changed at least once, but ideally twice daily.

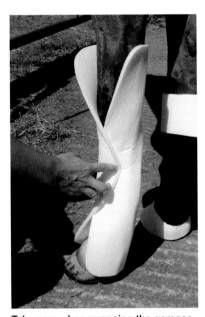

Take care when wrapping the gamgee around the leg to have the overlap to one side and not over the tendons

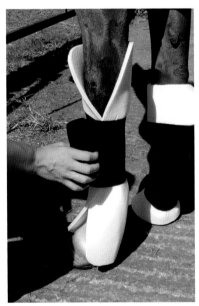

Apply the stable bandage using the same gentle, even pressure for the whole leg

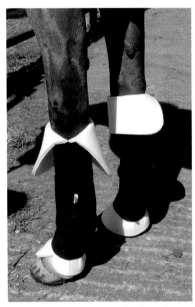

Stable bandages correctly placed on the front legs so the bandage extends from below the fetlock to just below the knee (or hock on the back leg)

BANDAGING AND POULTICING THE HOOF

FIRST AID FACTS

Puncture wounds (picture 1) and foot abscesses that cause pus in the foot and need draining will generally need bandaging and poulticing.

Remember that it is particularly important if your horse is lame on one leg to ensure that a supportive bandage is put on the opposite leg to prevent subsequent strain or injury to that leg.

WHAT YOU WILL NEED

- Flat dish to soak the poultice in
- Kettle, or other hot water source
- Optional iodine
- Poultice cut to size, e.g. Animalintex™
- Bucket of clean water and scrubbing brush
- Antiseptic solution
- Self-adhesive bandage e.g. Vetrap™
- Hard-wearing tape e.g. Ducktape™
- Scissors

HOW TO DO IT
Poulticing

- Pre-prepare the poultice:
  - Cut the poultice to the correct size i.e. to cover the injured area (picture 2)
  - Soak it in hot water (with or without iodine) and have it close by.

- Clean the wound and the surrounding area thoroughly with an antiseptic solution, and use the scrubbing brush if necessary.
- Apply the poultice, plastic side away from the skin, soft side against the skin.
- Ensure that no part of the hot poultice comes into contact with any sensitive areas of the body – for example, the sensitive bulbs of the heel.

Bandaging the poultice over the foot

- Hold the poultice in place and cover the whole of the base of the foot, heels and hoof wall with self-adhesive bandage (picture 3).
- Fix the foot bandage in place with a hard-wearing tape (pictures 4 and 5).
- Note: For any other part of the body you will only need to use an adhesive bandage and will not have to apply the hard-wearing tape.

WHAT ELSE DO YOU NEED TO KNOW?

A poultice should be checked and changed at least once, but ideally twice daily. Once most of the discharge has been drained into the poultice, then dressing changes can be less frequent.

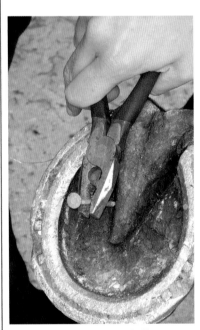

1 Remove any foreign body if necessary, and then mark the affected area

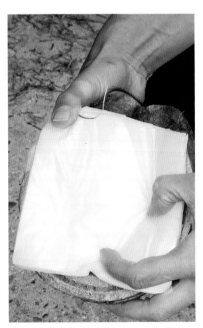

2 Place the soaked poultice into the foot, taking special care not to scald the heels

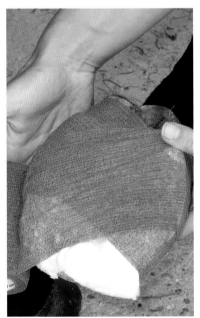

3 Secure the poultice in place with a self-adhesive bandage

POULTICING OTHER PARTS OF THE BODY

Other areas of the body can also be poulticed, and basically it is up to you to be as clever as possible in securing the poultice! Adhesive bandage, such as Polster Plast™, is ideal for use on areas other than the legs. For advice on how to secure a bandage on the legs, *see* Bandaging the Lower Leg (page 26).

For applying a poultice to parts of the body where you cannot secure a bandage to hold it in place – such as against an abscess in the neck, or an infected wound on the body – you can use a more hands-on approach. This requires you to hold a hot poultice against the affected area for 10 to 15 minutes two or three times a day.

For this hot poultice you can use anything that will hold heat, including a small hot-water bottle, a microwavable heat bag or a large glove containing a mix of bran and hot water.

Poulticing like this works by encouraging blood flow to the affected area, bringing more of the body's own infection-busting cells, and if the horse is on antibiotics, improving the blood flow improves exposure of the area to the antibiotics.

Usually an abscess or infected wound will come to a head, rather like a large spot, and then burst open. This looks much worse than it is, because once the infection has been drawn out, healing will be much quicker. You can then stop poulticing and treat it as an open wound.

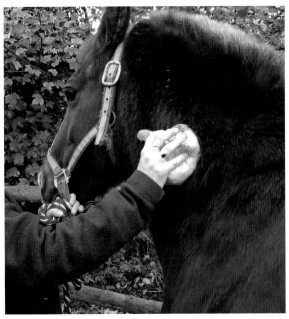

Use a soft, malleable heat source against a swelling to help draw infection out

TOP TIP

If the poultice becomes uncomfortably hot to hold, then it is also uncomfortable for the horse, so allow it to cool slightly before continuing.

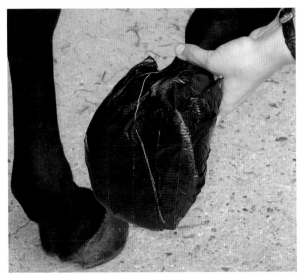
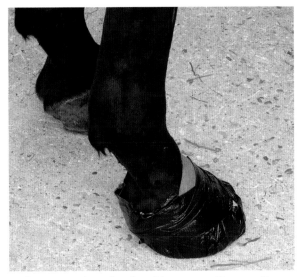

4 + 5 Hard-wearing tape can be used to make the poultice more robust: several overlapping strips are used to cover the sole of the foot and are then folded around the hoof; these ends are then secured in place when the foot is replaced on the floor

BANDAGING FOR LAMINITIS AND BRUISED SOLES

FIRST AID FACTS
'Cotton wool slippers' describes a way of bandaging the hoof that will give support and improve comfort for your horse if there is inflammation in the sole or hoof laminae. These slippers should only be used in mild cases; more severe cases will require proprietory frog supports fitted by the farrier or vet.

WHAT YOU WILL NEED
- Roll of cotton wool
- Self-adhesive bandage
- Hard-wearing tape
- Scissors

HOW TO DO IT
Pad the foot around the frog with cotton wool, then put a layer over the whole sole including the frog.

Hold the cotton wool in place with a layer of self-adhesive bandage, and fix this in place with a hard-wearing tape.

WHAT ELSE DO YOU NEED TO KNOW?
This type of bandaging should be kept on until the pain subsides. The bandages only need to be changed if the foot gets wet or damp, or if they begin to fall off.

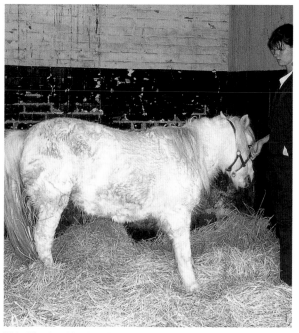

This Shetland is showing a typical laminitic stance, leaning backwards to ease the foot pain; careful bandaging of the feet to support the frog and sole of the foot will help to relieve the discomfort

---

BANDAGING THE LOWER LEG

FIRST AID FACTS
The aim of dressings in this situation is to protect the wound from further contamination, and to speed healing.

> **TOP TIP**
>
> Have all your bandages ready and within easy reach before you start dressing the wound.

WHAT YOU WILL NEED
- Hosepipe or bucket of clean water and large syringe
- Antiseptic solution
- Swabs or cotton wool
- Wound dressing e.g. Melonin™
- Padding bandage e.g. Soffban™, Orthoban™
- Conforming bandage e.g. K-band™
- Self-adhesive bandage e.g. Vetrap™
- Adhesive bandage e.g. Elastoplast™
- Scissors

HOW TO DO IT
Cleaning the wound
- Flush the wound thoroughly with plenty of clean fresh water to wash out any debris.
- Once you are happy the wound is free of dirt, then clean it with antiseptic solution, either chlorhexidine (Hibiscrub™) or iodine (Povidine™).
- If you have gauze swabs in your first aid box, you should use these rather than cotton wool as they leave fewer fibres in the wound.
- Dry the area around the wound thoroughly.
- Apply the wound dressing to the injury, ensuring the whole wound is covered.

> **TOP TIP**
>
> The padding layer is the most important part of the bandage as it holds the dressing in place and protects the underlying tissue from further damage.

Bandaging the wound

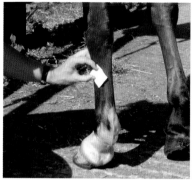

1 Choose a dressing that comfortably covers the wound all the way round

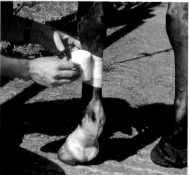

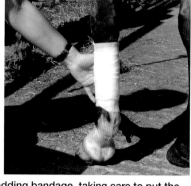

2 + 3 Secure the dressing in place with padding bandage, taking care to put the bandage on firmly but not too tightly

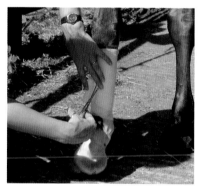

4 Next apply the conforming bandage: the aim of this is to secure the padding to the leg in a smooth layer that will not slip

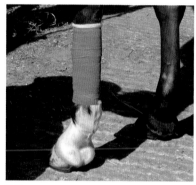

5 Now put on the self-adhesive bandage, to protect the underlying bandage. Be careful, as it is easy to put it on too tightly

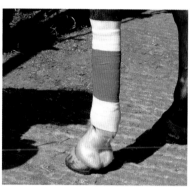

6 To help prevent the self-adhesive bandage slipping, adhesive bandage can be applied at the bottom and top

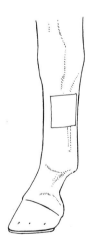
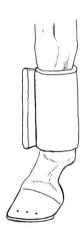
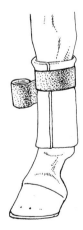
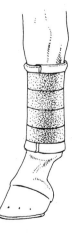

This sequence clearly illustrates the basic layers of bandaging for the canon. First ensure the dressing is covering the whole wound, and follow with a thorough layer of padding. The supporting layers of conforming and self adhesive bandages are traditionally applied from front to back around the leg to form a smooth even layer

WHAT ELSE DO YOU NEED TO KNOW?

The dressing and bandaging should be changed every two to three days, or as your vet directs – heavily discharging wounds will need redressing more frequently.

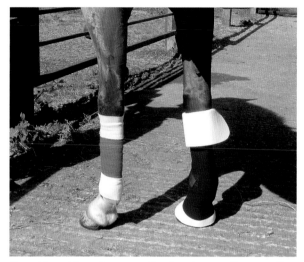

Do not forget to put a supporting bandage on the opposite limb to the injury

BANDAGING THE KNEE OR HOCK

FIRST AID FACTS

Once you are certain that the joint capsule has not been involved in the wound – if you are in any doubt check with your vet – then you can apply a bandage in the same manner as for the lower limb. Special care must be taken to prevent the bandage being too tight over the prominent parts of the joint; extra padding can be used, or releasing incisions made in the bandage.

HOW TO DO IT

Bandaging the carpus (knee)

At the back of the knee is the accessory bone, a 2–3cm (¾–1in) protrusion from the back of the knee.

KEEPING BANDAGES IN PLACE

Both knee and hock bandages are difficult to keep in place as there is so much movement in this part of the body: the use of adhesive tape at the top and bottom of these dressings can help to anchor the bandage in position. This can be further helped by putting extra turns of the foundation parts of the bandage around the less mobile parts of the leg above and below the joint.

Once these bandages are in place, a stable bandage can also be put on to help support the leg and keep the bandage edges clean.

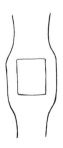 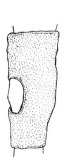 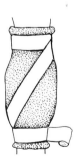 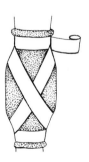 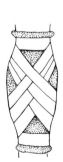 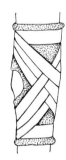

The most important factor in bandaging the knee is to ensure that there is not too much pressure applied over the accessory carpal bone. A figure-of-eight pattern of application for the supporting layers allows the bandage to be held in firmly in position without producing undue pressure on the delicate structures of the knee

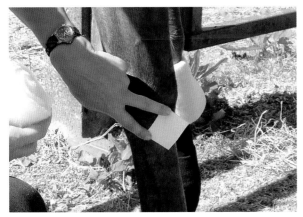
1 Choose a suitable dressing to cover the wound

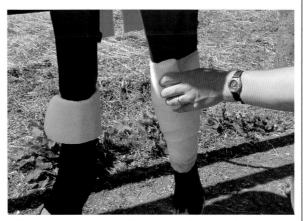
2 When applying the padding layers of the bandage, extra layers should be used over the accessory bone

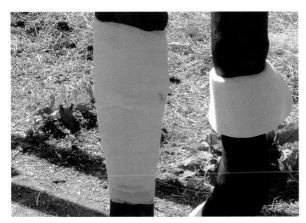
3 Ideally use a figure-of-eight pattern with the cross-over in the front of the knee to build up some padding on each side of the accessory bone before applying further padding over the whole area

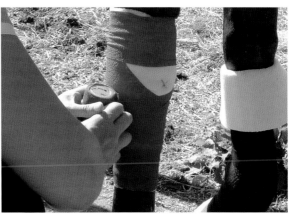
4 When the self-adhesive bandage is applied, try to avoid bandaging over this area until the last minute so there is very little pressure on the bone

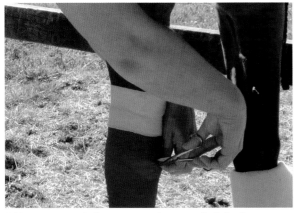
5 If you are worried, you can make a small slit in the outer bandage directly over the accessory bone. Secure with adhesive tape

WHAT IS SCAR TISSUE, AND HOW CAN IT BE MINIMIZED?

Scar tissue is produced in areas where healing has been slow or difficult. Scar tissue is weaker than healthy skin: a year after an injury the scar tissue at the site will have only 80 per cent of the strength of healthy skin. This is because the collagen produced in the healing process is weaker than the collagen found in normal skin, though over time this weaker collagen is replaced. Scarring can be minimized by careful attention to the wound to encourage rapid healing.

Bandaging the hock

The point of the hock is the area at risk with this bandage; furthermore it is a difficult part of the leg to keep a bandage on.

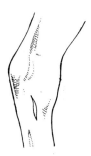
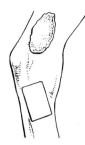
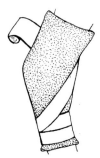

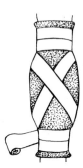
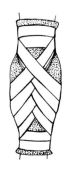
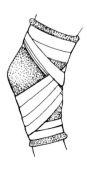

30

To help keep the bandage above the hock from slipping, pad the groove either side of the gastrocnemius tendon as this will help give a firm base to build the bandage on. Using a figure-of-eight pattern of application for the supporting layers will hold the bandage securely without putting pressure on the point of the hock

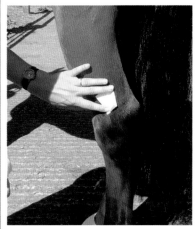

1 Choose a suitable dressing to cover the wound

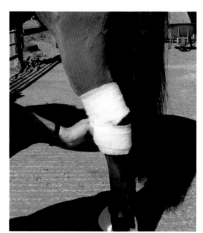

2 Apply the padding bandage: depending on the size of your horse, you may find it necessary to pad the grooves just above the point of the hock and below the *gastrocnemius* (Achilles) tendon, as this can help to fill out the bandage and stop it slipping

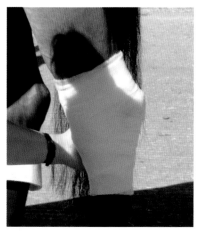

3 Next apply the conforming bandage: as with the carpus, a figure-of-eight pattern is useful to avoid covering the point of the hock until the last minute

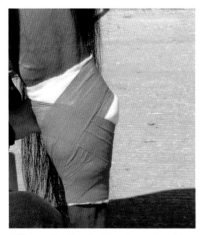

4 The self-adhesive bandage should also use the figure-of-eight pattern to fix the bandage firmly above and below the hock, again only covering the point of the hock at the last minute

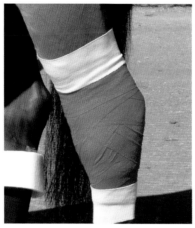

5 Secure with adhesive tape

WHAT CAN GO WRONG?

Over-tight bandages can cause serious damage to the leg underneath, cutting off the circulation and in serious cases damaging the underlying skin and tendons; these may then require surgical repair or long-term dressings.

Loose bandages that slip or wrinkle will also risk causing damage to underlying tissues, because they tend to move to an area where they are too tight, when they will inhibit the circulation.

Dressings that are not changed frequently enough can encourage infection and cause complications in wound healing. Also, dressings that become contaminated by bedding material or muck working up underneath can cause further injury to the skin and wound.

BANDAGING UPPER LIMBS

Getting bandages to stay put higher up on the limbs can be very difficult because the leg is wider at the top than at the bottom. However, this can be counteracted by increasing the padding around the leg to make it a more uniform tubular shape. The extra padding also allows you make the outer layers slightly tighter giving more grip.

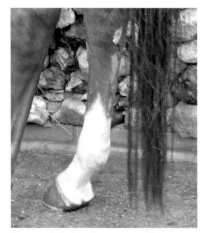

An overtight bandage on this leg rubbed the hair from the back of the canon. It was lucky this was noticed early: if this bandage had been left longer there may have been more substantial damage

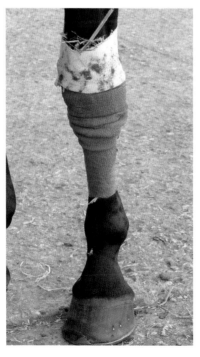

TOP TIP

If you are having problems keeping straw or dirt out of a bandage you can use a large tubular bandage in a double layer, stretched above and below the edges of the bandage and secured with adhesive tape.

This bandage has slipped considerably and risks putting pressure on the prominent accessory bone: it should be removed immediately

GETTING THE BEST FROM YOUR VET

HOW TO ACHIEVE THIS (IF YOU HAVEN'T ALREADY)

BARE FACTS

If you are choosing a new practice, work out what is important to you; for example:

- the cost of visits;
- how far ahead you need to book a routine appointment;
- whether the practice carries out equine dentistry, and to what level;
- how advanced the practice is (that is, whether it is a local mixed practice, a solely equine practice, or a specialized hospital);
- what facilities and equipment are available – x-rays, ultrasound, surgery, anaesthesia.

Write these questions down, and then phone your chosen practices and ask the questions.

TOP TIP

Your vet should not be scary to either you or your horse. Furthermore you should feel comfortable to phone your practice to speak to a vet or nurse for advice at any time.

If you are new to an area and not sure where to start choosing your new practice, ask other horse owners in the area for recommendations; most people are happy to tell you about both good and bad experiences that they have had with local practices.

If your horse is on a livery yard, find out which practice most people use and why; if you then go with that practice you may be able to share visit fees for routine procedures such as vaccination. Some practices have different levels of accreditation, depending on the facilities they have.

When deciding on a practice you must consider your expectations for both the performance of your horse, and how far you are likely to wish to take treatment. Some practices have more limited diagnositic, surgical or

nursing facilities then others, which is not generally a problem unless you have performance horses who tend to suffer from subtle lameness that requires experience and good diagnostic facilities in order to pinpoint the problem to allow a rapid return to competition.

Once you find a vet within the practice that you and your horse feel comfortable with, make sure you know their name and always ask for them; this way you have the opportunity to build a relationship with your vet, and they with you and your horse. It is a lot easier to make a diagnosis on vague symptoms if the vet already knows the patient and their little idiosyncrasies.

If your horse has a particular foible, then say so: no vet will appreciate being told that the horse doesn't

TOP TIP

Remember to tell the practice if your horse has a phobia to, say, men/women/ moustaches so they can send a suitable person to visit you. However, be aware that in an emergency your regular vet may not be available – though in an emergency this is not relevant.

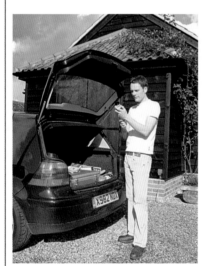

Both you and your horse should feel comfortable with your vet

like having its back legs handled once they've been kicked. Forewarned is forearmed, and will mean that the necessary steps can be taken to make the visit and treatment as quick, stress free and painless as possible for everyone involved.

If you are not comfortable with the way the vet is going about something, then SAY SO. Most horses have little tricks to make them easier to manage, so if you can see them doing something the horse hates, explain the situation, and it will mean less stress for everyone.

If you are unhappy with a vet, or something they have said or done, then again, SAY SO. Initially it is best

TOP TIP

If you don't like the vet or the practice, then vote with your feet and move. Everyone has different styles of working, and if theirs does not suit you, don't be afraid to move.

to speak to the vet directly as this can often lead to a satisfactory resolution. If, however, you are still unhappy, consult the practice manager, or go elsewhere. Serious complaints relating to malpractice can be taken up with the relevant regulatory body (in the UK, the Royal College of Veterinary Surgeons) .

Ask questions. If you don't understand, then ask, and ask again – if you understand the problem your horse has, you will be better able to nurse it and speed the recovery. If your mind always goes blank when the vet arrives (and then as they leave there are all those questions you thought of earlier…), write the questions down before the vet gets there, or phone them afterwards for clarification.

TOP TIP

You can ask for a second opinion on a medical condition without necessarily changing practices, or if you wish to explore other treatment options. Different vets have different approaches, and sometimes a fresh view on a condition can give a different line of enquiry; alternatively, it may simply confirm that the current approach is the most appropriate.

33

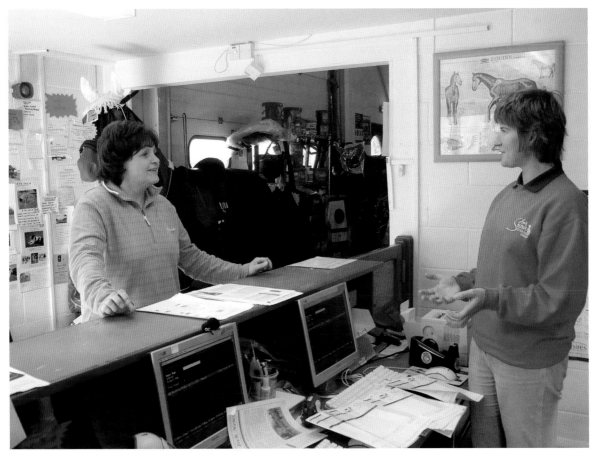

Helpful reception staff are an important part of a good veterinary practice

EUTHANASIA

BARE FACTS

This can be a difficult and emotive topic to discuss, and unfortunately few people think about it in advance. However, being aware of the different choices that may be available at such an emotional time can make the decisions easier. If you have an elderly horse with a chronic illness, while it may seem morbid, discussing the options and making your choices beforehand means that when the final moments arrive there is already a plan in place which can run smoothly, keeping the stress levels down for both you and your horse.

> **TOP TIP**
>
> The welfare of the horse has to be the primary consideration. This may appear to be stating the obvious, but at times of such distress it can be difficult to see what is the best course of action.

WHEN IS THE RIGHT TIME?

The first question that is usually asked is also one of the hardest to answer, and that is 'when is the right time?'. Sometimes there is little choice: if a horse is critically injured or ill, then your vet will explain there is no further treatment that will help it, and that a decision needs to be made there and then.

Old horses that are simply slowing down or struggling with arthritis, laminitis or teeth problems are more difficult. Often they have been having treatment over a prolonged period of time and the decline has been gradual, and this is the hardest decision to make. Some of the problem is that when you see an animal on a day-to-day basis you don't notice the gradual decline; in these circumstances the opinion of someone you trust outside the household can be invaluable.

Remember, your vet is on your horse's side: there is no vet who will suggest putting an animal to sleep if it is not truly in that animal's best interests. This is when time spent building a good relationship with your vet pays off.

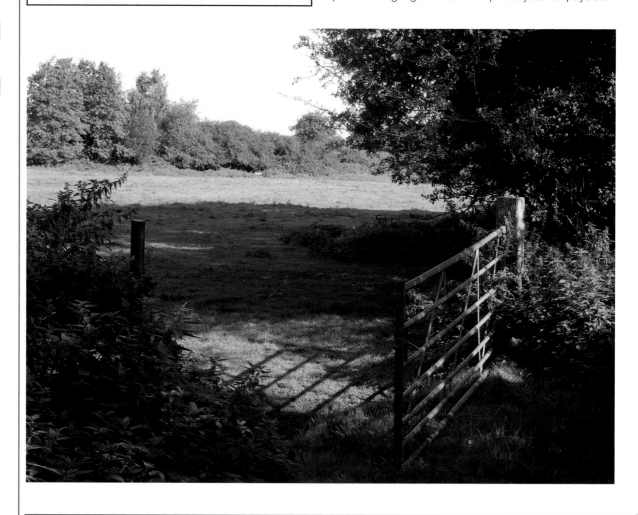

HOW SHOULD IT BE DONE?

The next decision you will have to make is whether to have an injection, or whether to have the horse shot. Many people already have clear views on this: it is a very personal decision, with no right or wrong answer. There are a few factors which may affect the decision, such as if you want your horse to go to the hunt kennels, then there can be no chemicals in the body which may poison the hounds, so shooting is the only option.

TOP TIP

If you have a horse that is severely 'needle-phobic' then it is worthwhile considering shooting, because if he has never seen a gun, then it is less likely to provoke a strong fear reaction.

LETHAL INJECTION

First, a strong sedative is injected into the vein, and given time to take effect – sometimes this will mean that the horse sways or lies down. Once the horse is settled, calm and comfortable, then a second, larger injection will be given into the vein. This is a massive overdose of anaesthetic drugs which makes the horse rapidly lose consciousness in exactly the same way as a general anaesthetic; then as the anaesthetic deepens, the breathing and then the heart stops. When this happens, if the horse is still standing it may topple suddenly, so if you have decided to hold the head while the injection is given, be very careful not to get trapped.

SHOOTING

A horse can be put down by shooting by your vet, the local huntsman or the knackerman. It will need to be done in a quiet area with as few people around as possible; a bucket of feed is usually all that is required to keep the horse quiet. The person with the gun will give you instructions on how they prefer to have the horse held and positioned, and then when everything is under control the barrel of the gun will be placed on the forehead and the trigger pulled. Collapse and death is instant: the bullet travels faster than the nerves can send pain signals, so the horse feels nothing. There is usually some bleeding from the bullet hole and from the nostrils, and there will often be some muscle spasms, but these are not conscious movements.

A common reflex post mortem is a gasping movement, known as an **agonal gasp** or **agonal breathing**, which can happen up to an hour after death. This is seen more commonly in older animals, and can happen whichever method of euthanasia is chosen. It is a reflex movement that only happens once the heart is stopped and the horse has died, and it should not be mistaken for the animal trying to breathe or recover.

WHERE SHOULD THE BODY GO?

The final decision is what to do with the body afterwards; this matter has been complicated recently by changes to the law regarding burying livestock, which includes horses. While it is illegal to bury livestock, guidelines have been issued which allow some leniency for horses, but the exact interpretation varies between individual councils. If your council is not horse friendly, or if you do not have the space, then the horse can go either to the kennels, or to the knackerman, or for cremation.

The hunt kennels will often collect and remove the body with no charge, or for a small handling fee; the knackerman will charge for collecting and dealing with the body, and this varies according to the distance he needs to travel, to where he is taking the body. Finally, some pet crematoriums collect and cremate horses (even Shire horses), and you may be able to have the ashes back; though obviously this can cost quite significantly more than the other options. Again, there is no wrong decision, only what you feel comfortable doing.

MINIMIZE STRESS

There are a number of different decisions that need to be made when the time comes, and experience has shown that a very difficult day can be made easier to bear if some thought and planning has gone into this whole matter beforehand. If *you* are less distressed, then your horse will be less stressed, and that has to be a good thing for everyone.

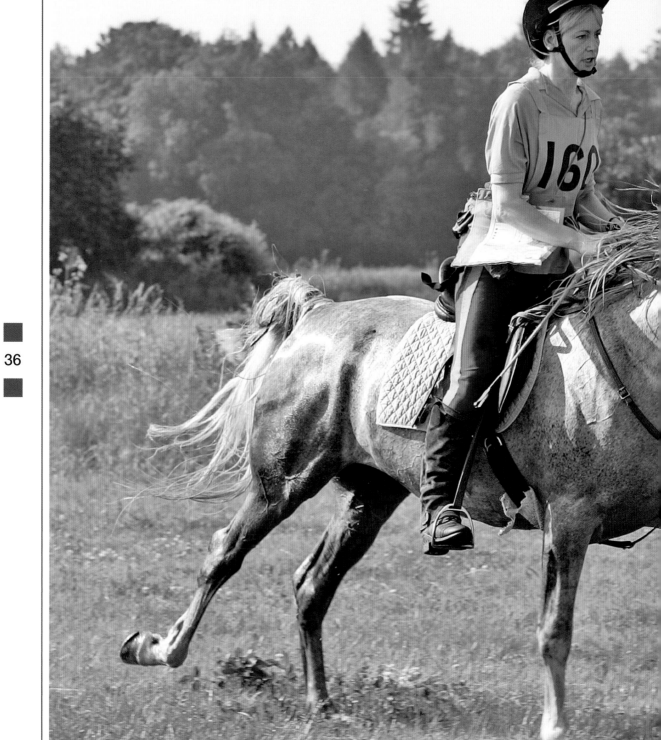

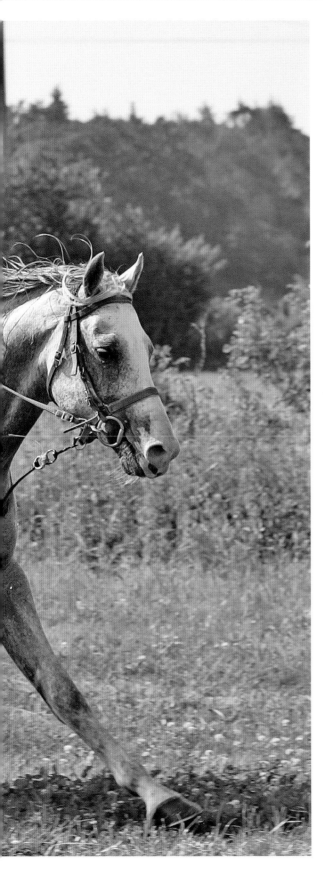

SECTION 2
OVERVIEW
OF THE BODY
SYSTEMS

This section works systematically through the basic organ systems which make up the horse, explaining for each the health problems that you may encounter and the first aid needed to help you cope with them – and when it is important to call for professional advice and assistance. Some common first aid myths are also discussed.

BONES

THE BARE BONES

The horse skeleton consists of, on average, 205 bones: it has 18 pairs of ribs, there are 34 bones in the skull, and each leg has 20 individual bones. Injury to the bones and joints is comparatively rare, but when it does occur, veterinary advice should be sought immediately.

Signs of a healthy skeleton
- Clean lines with no bumps, lumps, heat or swelling.
- No pain when moving.
- No restriction in the movement of the limbs.

Injuries to the skeleton
- Joint injury (injury within the joint capsule).
- Broken bones, including fracture of the skull.

JOINT INJURY

FIRST AID FACTS

Joint capsule injury is usually caused by an unlucky puncture wound, most commonly as a result of a fall on the road, or because the horse has become entangled in barbed wire. The most commonly affected joints are the pastern, fetlock, knee and hock joint, as these are the joints where the capsule is closest to the surface.

If a joint becomes infected it is known as **septic arthritis**: it becomes extremely painful very quickly (within hours of the infection being introduced), and there may be swelling around the joint or discharge from the wound.

Septic arthritis is a very serious condition needing expert and radical treatment as quickly as possible. However, it is not always treatable, and the welfare of your horse must be of first priority. Your vet will advise you whether you need to consider euthanasia.

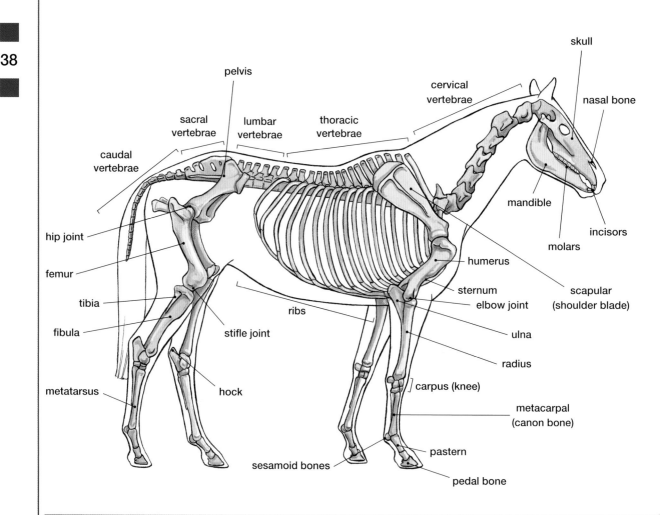

WHAT TO LOOK FOR

- You should look carefully for a puncture wound, a knock, or a strike injury near a joint. There may be swelling around the joint, or even pus coming from it.
- Once infection develops the horse will be in pain, often severe pain, and is likely not to be putting any weight on the affected limb.

WHAT TO DO

- Call your vet immediately for advice, explaining clearly what you see, and your horse's symptoms – and if you feel that your horse needs immediate veterinary attention, say so.
- Try and keep your horse calm and quiet; keeping movement of an injured joint to a minimum helps to reduce further damage.
- Use a rug to maintain his body temperature; this will help to keep him as comfortable as possible, and it will also slow the potential onset of shock.
- Use stable bandages to support his other, unaffected limbs and prevent further injury.
- Once you have spoken to your vet and know if specialist treatment is likely to be necessary you can organize transport to take your horse to the clinic or hospital as quickly as possible.

WHAT YOUR VET MAY DO

The initial examination will help determine if the joint capsule has been punctured or damaged; close inspection of the wound will help to clarify this. If any doubt, x-ray contrast can be injected into the joint: when an x-ray is taken, any leaks from the joint capsule caused by damage will show up clearly. If there is no joint capsule damage the wound will be treated as a simple laceration or puncture.

If it is a treatable injury the horse will be admitted to a veterinary hospital for a joint flush and capsule repair under heavy sedation or general anaesthetic. This involves flushing large volumes of sterile saline through the joint and the use of very high doses of antibiotics. The horse will need hospitalization to continue intensive treatment; however, if after repeated flushes the infection or pain does not resolve, then the vet will advise euthanasia.

WHAT CAN GO WRONG?

Untreated joint infections will cause severe acute lameness and irreversible joint damage. Furthermore, even if they are treated quickly and aggressively, some joint infections do not respond to therapy – and any time delay between the introduction of infection and the start of treatment decreases the chances of treatment being effective.

When infection is present, large volumes of sterile saline – sometimes containing antibiotics – are flushed through the joint. The initial procedure is usually performed under general anaesthetic, but once the apparatus is in place it may be repeated under standing sedation

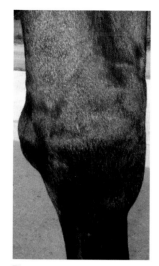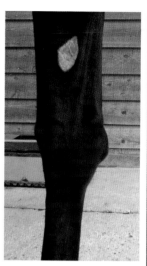

The uneven shape of this knee is the result of an OCD lesion which did not respond to aggressive treatment. Despite this deformation the horse is still ridable, but unable to compete at a high level

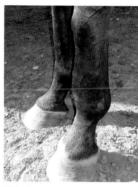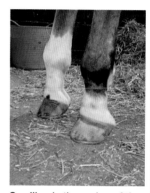

This former racehorse broke its canon bone when it was very young; surgical treatment was successful, however, and although the leg shape is abnormal, this horse has a normal life and is ridden regularly

Swelling in the region of the joint and refusing to weight bear on the limb is strongly suggestive of a serious injury to the joint capsule and should be treated as an emergency

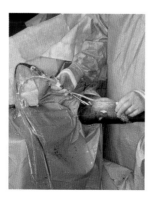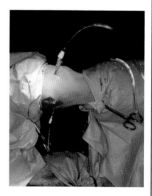

BROKEN BONES

FIRST AID FACTS

Broken bones are unusual in the horse. The long-term outcome depends on which bone is affected: a fracture of the skull, a rib, certain small bones within the knee or hock and some of the small bones of the foot can usually be treated.

The splint bone – an evolutionary remnant found on the inside of the cannon bone just under the knee – can be damaged by a kick from other horses, or by stress caused by exercise. It is painful, but usually recovers with rest, although some cases may require surgery to remove any detached fragments.

A break in one of the long bones of the leg carries a very poor prognosis, and usually euthanasia is the only humane option.

'Old Wives'Tales'

'MYTH':
A broken leg is a death sentence.

VET'S REPLY:
A break in one of the larger bones is very difficult to treat successfully as the size and weight of the animal involved can be greater than the pins and plates currently available are able to withstand. This means that although lower limb (the knee or hock and below) fractures in some cases may be able to be repaired surgically, you should be aware that there is a risk that even if your horse can have surgery to repair a fracture, there is always a risk that during recovery from the anaesthetic your horse can injure itself more severely.

WHAT TO LOOK FOR

- You may hear a loud crack.
- The horse refuses to put the affected limb to the ground.
- The limb may appear to be unstable or a different shape to normal.
- An **open fracture** is when the broken end of the bone is sticking through the skin – this is a hopeless case.
- The horse will be distressed at being unable to move normally, and in pain.
- In some cases the acute pain reaction does not seem to take effect immediately, but reaches its full impact after 10 to 20 minutes.

WHAT TO DO

- Call your vet immediately for advice. Be sure that you explain clearly what has happened to your horse: it may be easier for a friend to do this for you if your horse is very distressed. If you feel that your horse needs immediate veterinary attention you should not be afraid to say so.
- Try and keep your horse as quiet as possible: the less an injured limb is moved the better. A haynet is often the best way to distract a horse.
- Rug your horse up immediately: this will keep him warm and prevent the effects of shock developing.
- Bandage the unaffected limbs with stable bandages, to provide warmth and support.
- Having spoken to your vet, you should know if there is a probability of hospitalization for further treatment: organize transport so that your horse can be moved for treatment as soon as possible after the vet has examined the injury.

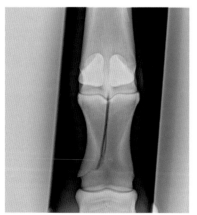
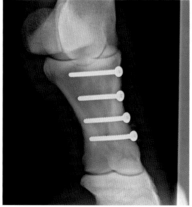

This fracture to the pastern bone has been repaired with the use of long surgical screws that will hold the bone fragments together until healing occurs. This fracture extends into the fetlock joint so there is a risk of this horse developing arthritis in the joint when it is older

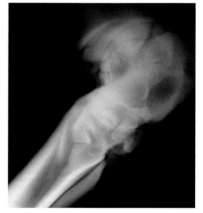

A fracture within a complex joint such as the hock holds a hopeless prognosis

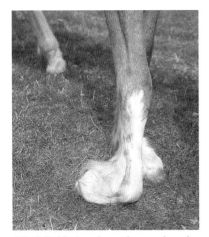

A limb held at such an abnormal angle is strongly suggestive of a fracture

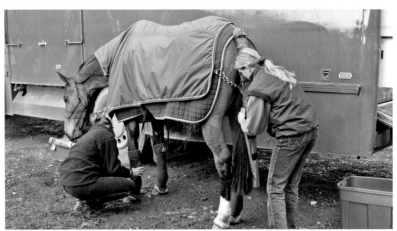

Any horse with a serious injury will be suffering from a degree of shock, so careful supportive bandaging, together with rugging up to maintain warmth, is important in maximizing its chance of recovery

WHAT YOUR VET MAY DO

The initial examination will involve palpation of the affected limb combined with an assessment of the general condition of the horse, and any other injuries which may have occurred at the same time and which will contribute to the outcome. If the injury is obvious and irreparable, then an immediate recommendation for euthanasia will be made.

Where there is either a question over the exact nature of the injury, or the appropriate treatment of the injury, then an x-ray will be taken. Most vets have portable X-ray machines, so this can usually be done without needing to move the horse very far. Once the x-rays have been taken, if treatment is likely to be undertaken, then a heavy-duty bandage (such as a Robert Jones bandage) or a splint will be applied to stabilize the limb and prevent further injury.

The treatment will be based on the radiographic appearance of the injury; in some cases this will involve surgery in order to stabilize the fragments of bone with plates and screws. Some minor fractures can heal with strict rest, depending on the site of the injury and the temperament of the horse.

WHAT CAN GO WRONG?

Fractures of long limb bones above the knee are rarely repairable in horses because of the strength of pull from the muscles and tendons is stronger than the surgical implants that are currently available to stabilize broken bones.

Furthermore the horse's efforts to get to his feet when recovering from general anaesthesia to repair one injury can result in severe injury to another limb, or serious muscle damage.

THE ROBERT JONES BANDAGE

The Robert Jones is a very thick, heavy-duty bandage with the supportive ability of a splint or a cast; it is often used to stabilize a limb immediately following an injury, prior to its definitive treatment, to allow the injured animal to be moved without exacerbating the injury. It involves applying a dressing over any breaks in the skin, followed by a thick layer of cotton wool closely conforming to the shape of the limb. This is then covered with layers of conforming bandage to gradually increase the tension in the bandage until when flicked with a finger, it sounds like a ripe melon. This layer is then covered with self-adhesive bandage to secure it. This is a very specialist bandage, and in order for it to be effective, it should only be applied by a veterinary professional.

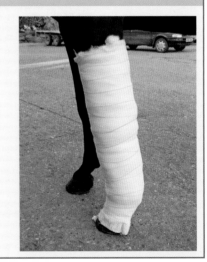

SKULL FRACTURES

FIRST AID FACTS

Skull fractures are rare, and are nearly always very painful. The bones of the skull are extremely strong and usually it requires a puncture-type injury to cause a fracture. A heavy fall can occasionally split the lower jaw at the point of the chin (*mandibular symphysis*) where the two halves of the lower jaw are fused.

If you think that the outline of the skull has lost its symmetry, or that part of it is moving in an abnormal way, then contact your vet immediately.

WHAT TO LOOK FOR

- If your horse has received a blow to the head strong enough to make you think there may be a fracture, call your vet immediately.
- If the jaw is affected there may be some instability in the teeth and an unwillingness to eat.
- If the bones of the skull are affected there is usually a depression over the site of the fracture which is painful to the touch.
- Some skull fractures can develop into painful, and occasionally hot, swellings.
- Injuries to the front of the face can damage the sinuses, leading to profuse bleeding from the nose.

WHAT TO DO

If you think your horse may have suffered a skull fracture, call your vet immediately.

WHAT YOUR VET MAY DO

X-rays will be needed to confirm that there is a fracture of the skull present. If this is confirmed, then depending on the severity and position of the fracture, surgical repair may be attempted. However, if the fracture has not displaced the bone, and it is not affecting the horse other than causing pain, then treatment may be restricted to pain relief while healing takes place.

WHAT CAN GO WRONG?

Fractures to the jawbone can inhibit eating, or may change the pattern of wear on the teeth, and this can result in the need for specialized feeding techniques and repeated dental treatment.

A complication is that fractures can introduce infection into the sinuses; these can become deep-seated, and are very hard to treat.

42

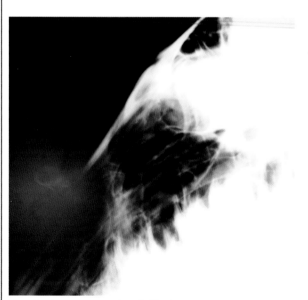

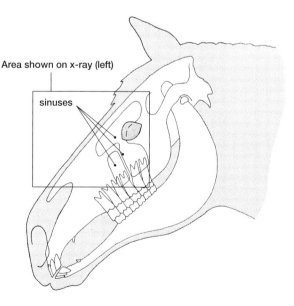

Area shown on x-ray (left)

sinuses

The sinuses are extensive air filled spaces within the skull, which are connnected to the nasal chambers. As can be seen from these illustrations the roots of some of the molars extend into these sinuses, this means that some dental conditions will show as a foul smelling nasal discharge as infection from the tooth root drains from the sinus into the nasal chambers and out through the nostril

SPLINTS

FIRST AID FACTS

The splint bone is an evolutionary remnant, known as a metacarpal in the front leg and a metatarsal in the back leg, that does not extend the full length of the canon bone. It serves no useful purpose.

The splint bone may be broken, or the ligament attaching it to the canon bone may be strained, and the thickening that is felt following this type of injury is referred to as a *splint*.

Sprains are most common in young horses that are being brought into heavy work, while fractures most commonly occur as a result of a direct blow – usually a kick or fall.

WHAT TO LOOK FOR

- The splint bone is most easily felt on the inside of the leg just below either the knee or the hock, although splint bones are also found on the outside of the leg.
- Injury to the splint bone can be caused either through stress – such as high levels of training – or by a direct blow such as a kick.
- An injured splint bone causes a degree of lameness, and there will be a firm, painful swelling over the point of injury.

WHAT TO DO

- If the lameness is mild, rest with supportive stable bandaging is usually sufficient for a sprain. If the lameness does not improve within a short time, seek advice.
- If the lameness is pronounced, and there is obvious swelling over the splint bone or there is a deep cut, call your vet for advice.

WHAT YOUR VET MAY DO

If there is no fracture to the splint, then supportive bandages, rest and pain relief will be all that is necessary. If there is a suspicion of a fracture, x-rays will be taken to confirm its nature. In cases where the splint bone has been broken but there is little displacement between the ends of the bone, the treatment is the same as for a sprain but for a more prolonged period.

Surgery is usually only necessary if the fragments of broken bone are unlikely to heal on their own, if the skin has been broken and bone has been exposed, or it is an old injury which is proving difficult to resolve.

WHAT CAN GO WRONG?

Injuries that result in a fracture of the splint bone may require surgery in order to remove the detached fragment (*sequestrum*).

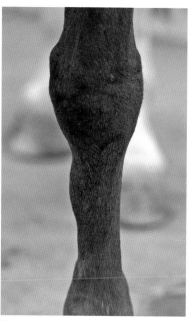

This leg shows a small splint swelling on the inside of the leg

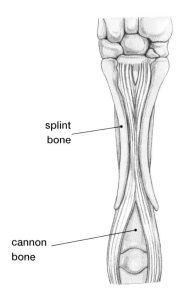

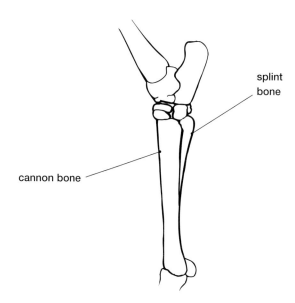

splint bone

cannon bone

splint bone

cannon bone

Splints can form all along the junction between the cannon and splint bone. The common site is on the medial (inside) side, roughly one third down the cannon

SPAVINS

FIRST AID FACTS

A 'spavin' is a disorder of the hock joint.

Bog spavin is an increase of fluid in the joint capsule of the hock, and is usually seen in younger horses.

Bone spavin is arthritis affecting the hock, and is usually seen in older horses.

WHAT TO LOOK FOR

- *Bog spavin* is a swelling on either side of the hock, towards the front of the leg, caused by too much fluid in the joint capsule; it is not normally painful, and does not cause lameness.
- *Bone spavin* causes lameness in the back leg; the lameness is worse when the hock has been fully flexed.

WHAT TO DO

- *Bog spavin* is primarily a cosmetic problem; however, similar symptoms can be caused by **osteochondritis dessicans** (OCD), so any swelling around the joint should be fully investigated.
- *Bone spavin* causes lameness because of the pain caused by the arthritic changes within the joint. Any chronic or recurrent lameness should be investigated.

WHAT YOUR VET MAY DO

A lameness work-up will include a trot-up to assess the affected limb and the degree of lameness; flexion tests can be used to confirm that the lameness is located in the hock. Local anaesthetic can be injected into the joint capsule to numb it – if the lameness improves dramatically after this technique, this can help to localize the cause of the pain more accurately.

X-rays will be taken from several different angles to check for the new bone growth of arthritis or cartilage damage caused by OCD. If there is suspicion of an infection or other inflammatory process causing the lameness – particularly if there is pain without changes on x-ray – then joint fluid samples can be taken for **cytology**.

- *Bog spavin*: as this is largely cosmetic, no treatment is usually necessary once other problems have been ruled out. If cosmetic appearance is important, the excess fluid can be drained and an injection given into the joint to discourage further fluid production.
- *Bone spavin*: depending on the severity of the condition, pain relief medication can be given, or long-acting steroids can be injected into the joint. More aggressive treatment includes surgical treatment to fuse parts of the joint.

WHAT CAN GO WRONG?

Bone spavin can cause irreparable damage to the hock joint, in the worst case scenario rendering the horse chronically lame, or at least reducing its degree of athletic ability and performance.

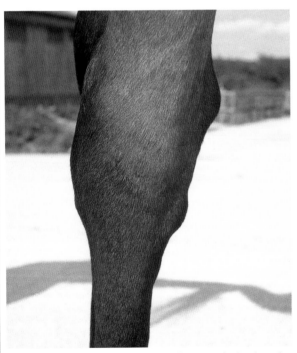
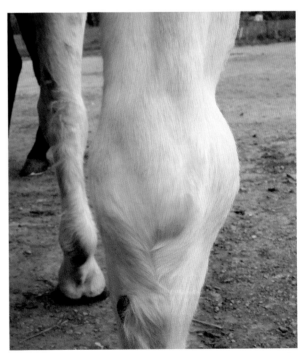

These pictures show abnormal swelling over the hock region, and both will require further investigation in order to ascertain the cause

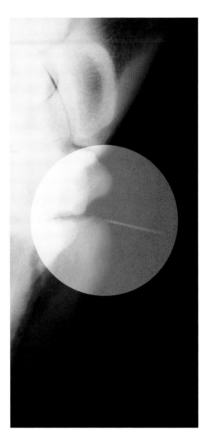

This x-ray of the hock illustrates the many articular surfaces present within the joint; the top of one of the splint bones is also highlighted

This x-ray of a hock shows a small probe which has been inserted into a wound on the back of the hock to investigate the depth of the wound, and assess if the joint capsule has been penetrated

WHAT IS A FLEXION TEST?

Flexion tests are performed as part of a lameness work-up or a pre-purchase examination, the aim being to highlight any underlying pain in a limb. This is achieved by picking the leg up as high as possible in order to stretch the joints, and holding this position for approximately 60 seconds. The horse is then led straight off into a trot, and the first few paces are watched very closely because if there is going to be lameness it is only in these first steps that it will be obvious. The flexion test can produce lameness in a horse that has appeared sound in the trot-up by stretching a joint and putting pressure on areas that are only used at exercise.

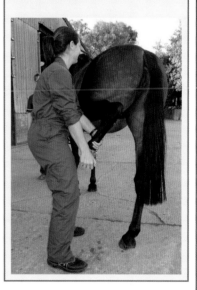

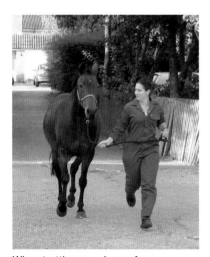

When trotting up a horse for a lameness assessment it is important to use a loose lead rein to allow for nodding of the head should he take any lame strides

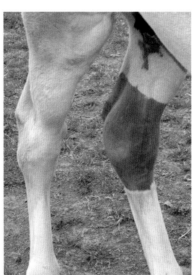

This hock has been clipped up to allow aseptic preparation of the skin prior to injection of medication into the joint

THE HEART, BLOOD AND CIRCULATION

THE BARE FACTS

The average horse's heart weighs approximately 10kg (22lb) and beats between 30 and 40 times a minute; at rest a horse's heart it pumps around 1ltr (1¾ pints) of blood per beat.

An average horse of 550kg (1,200lb) has approximately 45ltr (10gal) of blood in circulation; a 10 per cent blood loss (4.5ltr/1gal) can be easily balanced out by the body so that no ill effects are seen.

Signs of a healthy circulation:

- The gums and inside of the eyelids should be salmon pink in colour.
- If pressure is applied to the gums the colour should return within two seconds – this is termed the 'capillary refill' time.

- If the skin is pinched up between the fingers and then dropped, it returns to its normal position quickly; this can vary between horses, however, so find out what is normal for your horse – this is termed 'skin tenting'.
- The pulse is strong and regular.
- Quiet, calm breathing when the horse is at rest.
- No build-up of fluid around the body, especially under the abdomen.

Conditions affecting the circulation:

- Bleeding (damaged blood vessels) from wounds.
- Nosebleed.
- Shock.
- Heart attack.
- Blood in unusual places (in the faeces, or urine, or coughing up blood) may indicate a problem in the horse's system.

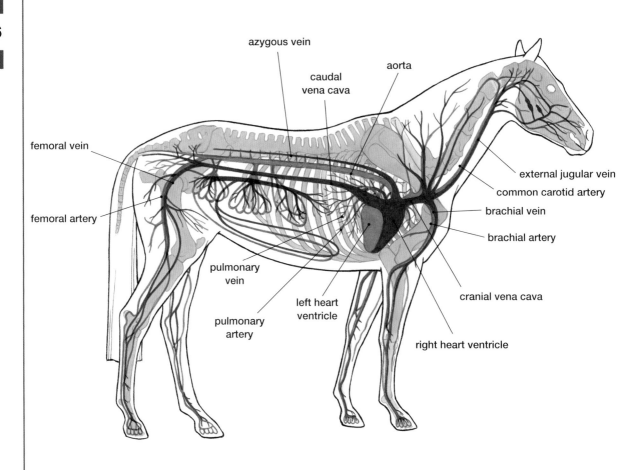

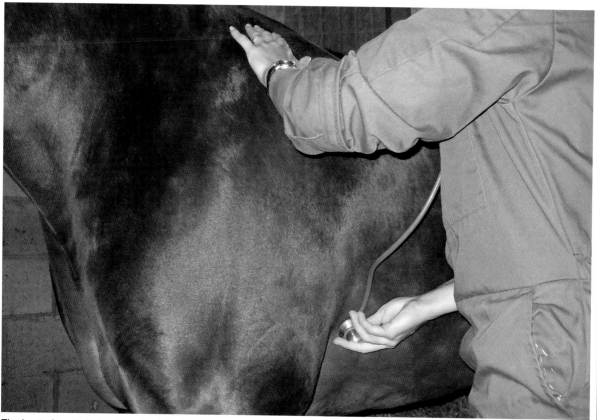

The best place to listen to, or feel the heartbeat, is just behind the left elbow

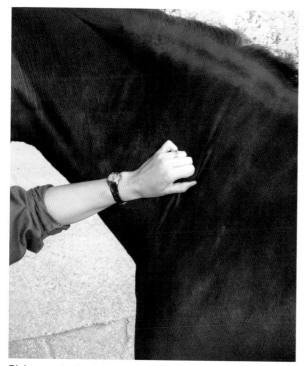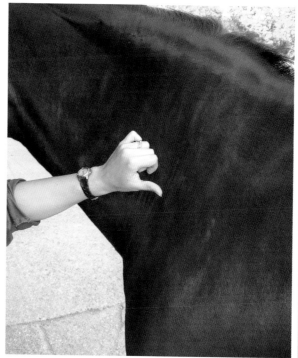

Pick up a pinch of skin on the point of the shoulder; when you let it go, it should drop down flat again within one to two seconds

BLEEDING WOUNDS

FIRST AID FACTS

If your horse has a bleeding wound, the colour of the blood and the pressure of the bleeding will usually indicate whether the injury is involving an artery or a vein, and how serious it is.

- An arterial bleed is bright red in colour and spurts at the same rate as the heart is beating.
- A bleed involving a vein tends to run or ooze and is a darker red.

The main arteries in the body are normally protected by their position in the body, usually running close to a bone and covered by a large muscle.

WHAT TO LOOK FOR

- Colour: arterial blood is brighter red than venous blood.
- Pressure: arterial blood will spurt in pulses, even from small arteries and arterioles, whereas blood from veins runs or dribbles without spurting.
- Speed: the bigger the vessel, the faster the blood flows, and the more important it is to control it.

WHAT TO DO

Blood from an artery

Bleeding that is bright red and spurting involves damage to an artery.

- Apply firm pressure on the site of the bleeding initially with your fingers, and…

- …ask someone to call your vet.
- If possible use an absorbent dressing or material to help slow the flow of the blood, and press as hard as you can.
- If it is still bleeding after a while and your fingers are aching, then a pressure bandage can be applied.

Blood from a vein

Bleeding that is darker red in colour, and is dribbling or oozing, involves a vein.

- A slow bleed can be controlled by using a dressing that is applied over the wound in order to provide some pressure.
- If the bleeding is more profuse, then an absorbent dressing can be held in place by hand in order to apply greater pressure.
- If the bleeding has not slowed down or stopped within 10 minutes, call your vet.

TOP TIP

A little blood can go a long way – remember that horses can lose a surprisingly large volume of blood with no obvious ill effects.

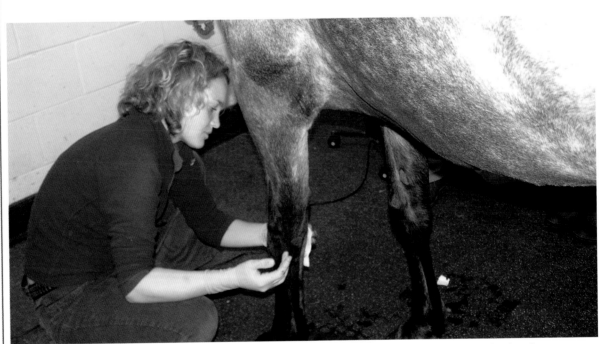

Laceration of even small arterioles can lead to a puddle of blood forming rapidly. It is important to maintain a firm pressure on the source of the bleeding until help arrives

'MYTH':
Bleeding a horse will help it run faster or relieve the symptoms of laminitis.

VET'S REPLY:
There is no scientific evidence to support this theory. It is based on the medieval practice of placing leeches to draw out bad blood. Top human athletes have been known to remove a pint of blood and store it, allowing their bodies to replace it; then just before an event they inject the removed blood back into their body to top up their levels of red blood cells to improve their oxygen-carrying capacity.

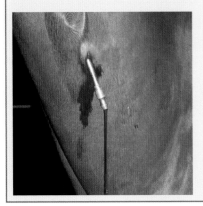

This racehorse is being bled because the trainer believes it will make it run faster in its next race

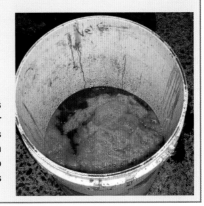

The bucket holds approximately 20ltr (4gal), and is half full; this demonstrates how much blood can be lost with no adverse effects

WHAT YOUR VET MAY DO
Wounds that bleed profusely often require surgery, under either general or local anaesthetic, to repair the injury and prevent further bleeding.

TOP TIP

If a bandage is used to control the bleeding but the blood starts to show through, put another layer over the top to increase the pressure being applied; this prevents the clot which is forming from being disturbed.

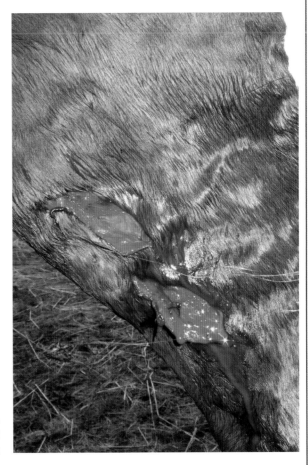

This wound is bleeding from damaged veins, as can be seen from the trickle of blood running down the leg

NOSEBLEEDS

FIRST AID FACTS

Nosebleeds (*epistaxis*) often look much worse than they are, and can continue for up to half an hour before stopping – although during this time the speed of the blood flow should become noticeably slower. A nosebleed can occur spontaneously, but is usually the result of a causal factor – such as during an examination when an endoscope or stomach tube is being passed through the nose and damages the tissues.

A nosebleed can also be caused by head trauma, such as might be incurred in a fall, or by a kick from another horse, or by hitting the head when rearing; or as a result of intensive exercise.

A very serious form of nosebleed can occur if your horse acquires a fungal infection of the **guttural pouch**, which is part of the sinus system in the head. A major artery passes through the guttural pouch, and it can be ruptured by a long-standing fungal infection. This is very rare, however, and before this stage is reached there are usually plenty of other clinical signs that will have been investigated, and which lead to a diagnosis and appropriate treatment.

WHAT TO LOOK FOR

- The colour of the blood: the darker it is, the slower the bleeding will be.
- The speed of the blood flow: this will indicate the severity of the problem – if you can count the drips, don't worry!

WHAT TO DO

- Do not try to obstruct the nostril(s) as horses cannot normally breathe through their mouth, and this will panic them.
- Put the horse somewhere quiet and allow them to settle on their own – hay is very good for this.
- Call your vet if the bleeding is not slowing down, or the blood is coming down both nostrils, or if the horse has had a series of nosebleeds.

WHAT YOUR VET MAY DO

There is little that can be done to stop a nosebleed. Once it has settled down, then the vet may examine the inside of the nose and airways using an endoscope to try and find the source of the bleed.

The most common finding of an endoscopic examination is a burst vessel in the sensitive folded tissues of the nasal cavities. If the nosebleeds keep recurring surgery can be performed to seal these bleeding vessels that lie high in the nasal cavity; this operation is usually performed at a referral hospital.

If the guttural pouch is the source of the bleeding, then the underlying problem must be identified. If there is a fungal infection (guttural pouch mycosis) then radical surgery can be attempted and topical treatment for the fungal infection started; however, this is a difficult condition to treat successfully.

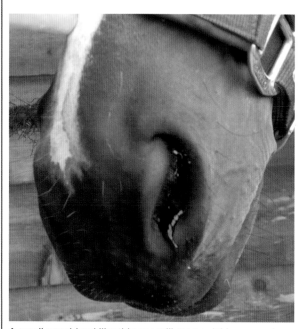

A small nosebleed like this one will stop quickly; you only need to call your vet if it recurs

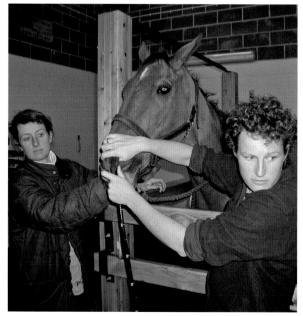

If nosebleeds persist then endoscopic evaluation of the upper airways will be performed to identify the problem

SHOCK

FIRST AID FACTS

Shock is a condition of the cardiovascular system, which occurs with very severe injury, loss of blood or an overwhelming infection. In shock, the normal regulation of the blood vessels is lost, and the blood is not directed around the body in an efficient manner. This will lead to the gums and conjunctiva changing from a healthy pink colour to pale pink or white, together with rapid breathing and shivering. The effects of shock are very similar to the symptoms felt by a person shortly before fainting.

WHAT TO LOOK FOR

You should look for any alterations from the signs of a healthy circulation; these alterations might include the following:

- The colour of the gums and around the eyes would be paler than the normally deep salmon pink.
- If pressure is applied to the gums the colour would be slower to return than the normal couple of seconds.
- A weak and irregular pulse.
- Rapid and shallow breathing.

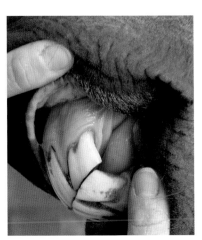 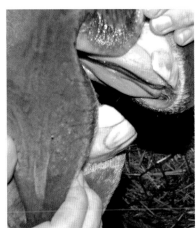 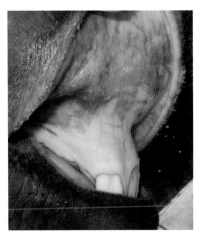

These are all normal healthy horses, and the photos serve to illustrate the differences in gum colour between individuals. Black pigment is a normal feature and should not be confused with colour changes caused by circulatory failure

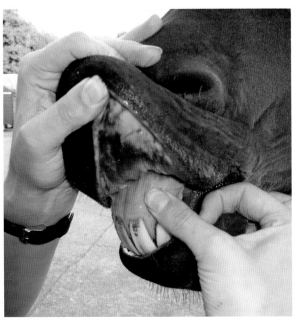 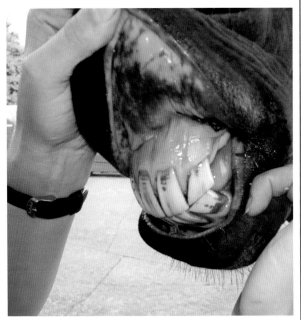

Testing capillary refill time: press hard on the gums for two to three seconds until the colour is blanched out, then release. The colour should return within two seconds

WHAT TO DO

- This is an emergency and your vet should be called immediately.
- The horse should be kept warm, and offered a warm drink, preferably an electrolyte solution.
- Do not try and move your horse, as the effects of shock will make it weak and therefore at risk of falling and injuring itself further.

WHAT YOUR VET MAY DO

In cases of severe shock the horse will be given very large volumes of intravenous fluids (20ltr (5gal)) as a rapid pulse to help support the cardiovascular system; he will be kept warm and quiet, and will be kept under very close observation by a veterinary professional.

The cause of the shock must be identified and treated; treatment may involve high doses of intravenous antibiotics, steroids or pain relief. If a focus of infection is discovered, then this will be treated aggressively to remove the source of toxins; this may involve surgery.

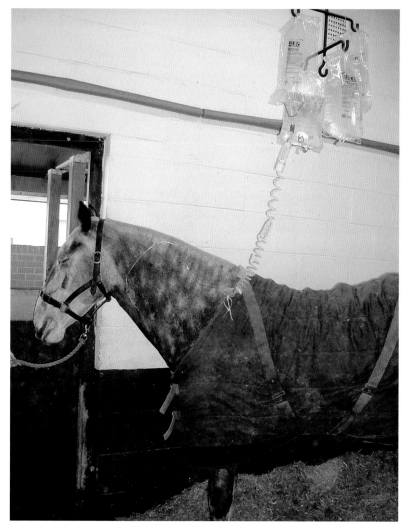

This horse is receiving intravenous fluids to support its circulation

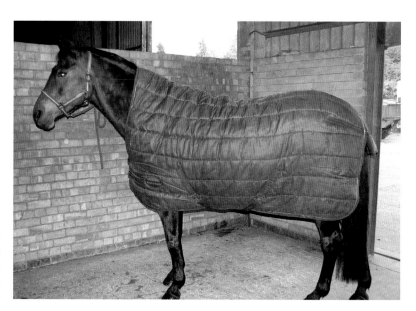

If you suspect your horse is suffering from shock, keep it warm to prevent its condition deteriorating, and seek veterinary advice

HEART ATTACK

FIRST AID FACTS

A heart attack in a horse is a rare event: it is caused by the heart muscles not receiving enough oxygen from their blood supply, which causes serious damage – as a result these muscles are not able to contract, and so the heart stops beating.

WHAT TO LOOK FOR

- Very rapid, shallow breathing.
- Ventral oedema.
- Disorientation.
- Sudden collapse.

WHAT TO DO

- This is an emergency: call your vet immediately.
- Try and keep your horse as calm as possible to prevent it panicking and causing further injury.
- Cover the horse with a rug to try to maintain body temperature and prevent the onset of shock.
- Do not make any attempt to move the horse, particularly if it has collapsed.

WHAT YOUR VET MAY DO

Usually a heart attack is fatal; if your horse survives the initial attack then appropirate supportive treatment may be given (*see* Shock, above) but sadly the most likely outcome is euthanasia.

Adrenalin can be administered to stimulate the heart to beat if it is failing, but for this to be effective it must be given very quickly after the heart attack, which is only likely to happen if a vet is immediately available and with the appropriate equipment to hand – really they would have to be standing in front of the horse at the time, the the adrenaline ready.

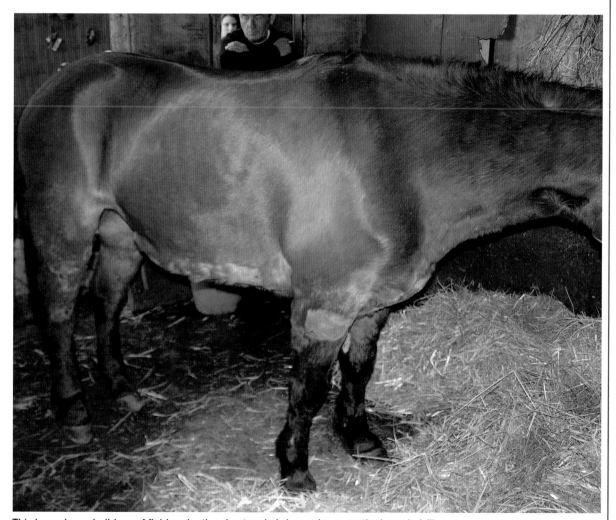

This horse has a build-up of fluid under the chest and abdomen because the heart is failing

BLOOD IN UNUSUAL PLACES

Blood should not be seen in:
• the faeces
• the urine
• the airways (if the horse were coughing up blood)

FIRST AID FACTS

If any amount of blood is seen in the faeces or the urine it is important to call your vet because it may suggest that a serious medical condition is developing.

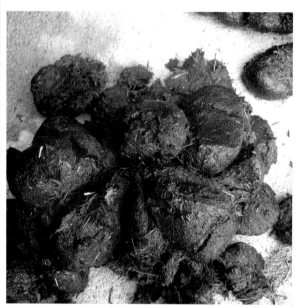

Blood around the droppings like this suggests there is some bleeding in the rectum

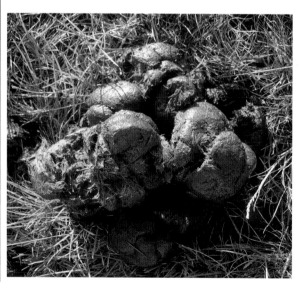

Normal, well formed droppings

Blood in the airways is normally caused by over-exertion at exercise and is therefore seen mostly in racehorses; however, it can be the result of chronic inflammation or infection in the airways.

WHAT TO LOOK FOR
Blood in the faeces/urine
■ Blood-red deposits that are mixed in with, or surrounding the faeces.
■ Black, tar-like faeces.
■ Darkened urine with a pink or red tinge, or blood splashes on the hind legs.

Coughing up blood
■ Streaks of blood in the saliva or nasal fluid.
■ Blood-stained mucus near water or food buckets.

WHAT TO DO
Blood in the faeces/urine
■ Call your vet.
■ Keep a sample of the affected urine or faeces as the vet may need it for analysis.

Coughing up blood
■ Rest your horse if you have been exercising it, and call your vet for advice straightaway.
■ Monitor your horse closely, and make a note of when you are seeing blood, and how much is present at any one time.

WHAT YOUR VET MAY DO
Blood in the faeces/urine
The vet will make a full physical examination of the horse; this may include a rectal examination or an ultrasound investigation of the abdomen. A blood sample is likely to be taken because this can show if there is infection, inflammation or a problem with one of the major organs, and a sample of the affected faeces or urine will also be tested.

If a problem is suspected with the last portion of the gut – the last metre approximately – biopsy samples may be taken and sent for histology.

Coughing up blood

A full physical examination of the horse will need to be made; this will include listening carefully to the chest and possibly the throat. It may also include close examination of the mouth, the **lymph nodes** (glands) of the face and neck, and endoscopic examination of the upper airways. Blood samples and samples of fluid from the airways may be taken for analysis to assess for levels of infection and inflammation.

If the bleeding is related to exercise, then endoscopic evaluation may be carried out after a period of intense exercise in an attempt to trigger some bleeding so the source can be located. Your horse may be referred to a sports medicine clinic for evaluation on a treadmill as this makes it possible to watch the airways with an endoscope while it is at full gallop.

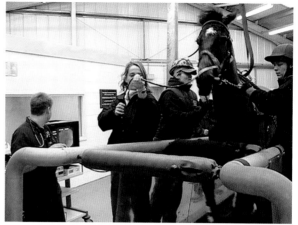

Some competition horses have small bleeds into the airway when they are exercising at a high level; this can be mimicked in a clinical environment with the use of an endoscope to examine the airways while the horse is worked at a gallop on a treadmill

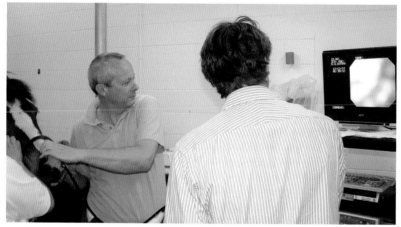

Recurrent nosebleeds can be investigated by endoscope; this allows visualization of the sensitive tissues of the upper nasal cavity as well as the guttural pouch

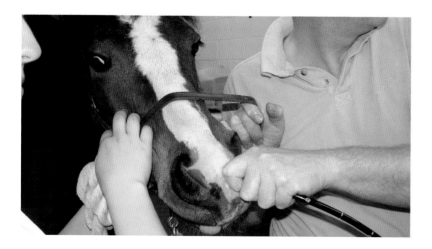

THE LUNGS AND BREATHING

THE BARE FACTS

The average horse takes 10 to 14 breaths per minute at rest, breathing in approximately 80 litres (18 gallons) of air each minute; this can increase to approximately 1,800 litres (400 gallons) per minute at a gallop.

The respiratory rate is a useful indicator of the health of the horse, increasing with fever and pain, and both rate and depth increase with exercise – the rate of recovery being a good indicator of fitness levels.

Signs of healthy airways

- At rest the breathing is quiet, slow and regular.
- No wheezing or coughing at rest or exercise.
- Clean dry nostrils with no discharge.

Conditions affecting the respiratory system

- Allergic airway disease (COPD/RAO).
- Nasal discharge.
- Equine flu and colds.
- Strangles.

EPIGLOTTAL ENTRAPMENT

Horses that are pushed to the extreme of their physical abilities, particularly racehorses, can suffer from a condition called *epiglottal entrapment*, in which the **epiglottis** becomes trapped out of its normal position and completely – albeit temporarily – blocks the airways. Racehorses can also suffer from small bleeds from their trachea. Both of these conditions are usually only exhibited under extreme physical stress.

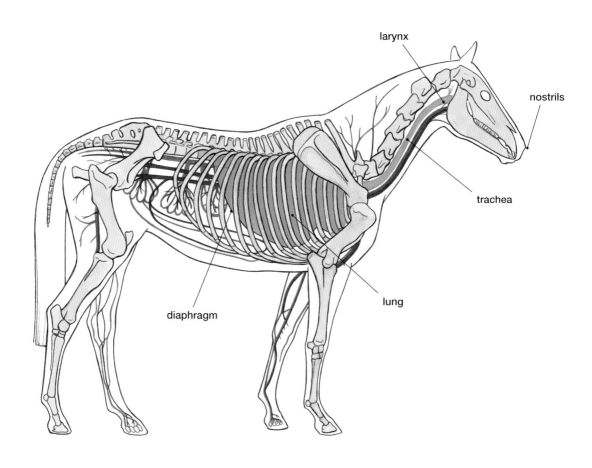

larynx

nostrils

trachea

lung

diaphragm

ALLERGIC AIRWAY DISEASE

FIRST AID FACTS

Allergic airway disease (COPD/RAO) is a problem most commonly seen in older horses and ponies. It is brought on by exposure to airborne irritants, in particular fungal spores and pollen. Exposure to these irritants can be reduced by good stable management – the use of low dust bedding such as shavings, the installation of good ventilation, and by soaking hay or feeding treated hay.

Often the symptoms are initially seasonal, but they will extend into the rest of the year as the condition develops and becomes more severe. If your horse suffers from this condition, then consult your vet for more specific advice on your stable environment, as controlling this will have a significant effect in reducing the symptoms.

WHAT TO LOOK FOR

- The horse will make more noise than should be normal during either inspiration (breathing in) or expiration (breathing out).
- There will be increased movement of the ribcage.
- A muscle line along the abdomen – known as the 'heave line' – will gradually develop.
- A persistent, clear watery discharge in both nostrils, which may become creamy or green if secondary infection develops.
- A persistent cough, even at rest.

WHAT TO DO

- Audible wheezing, often when the horse is stabled, is usually a sign of chronic obstructive pulmonary disease (COPD) or recurrent airway obstruction (RAO). Normally this is an allergic reaction, similar to asthma where the airways narrow because of swelling in response to the irritant.
- Changing the bedding to reduce dust, improving ventilation and soaking hay all reduce possible irritants. But if this condition continues, then call your vet.

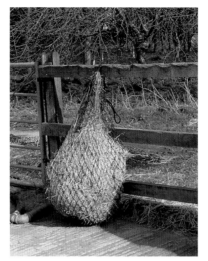
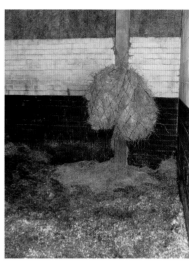

Soaking the haynet will help your horse's airways, but stable hygiene must also be maintained at a high level, unlike in this example at right

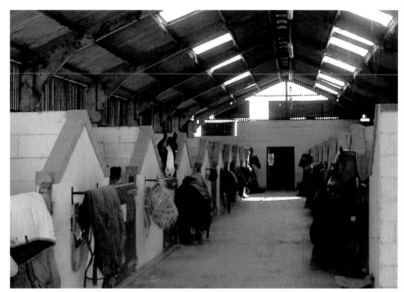

Barn stabling such as this has good ventilation, which prevents the build-up of dust and other contaminants in the atmosphere, contributing to good respiratory health in its residents

- Make sure your horse is taken away from the stable while you are mucking out so that all the dust and spores kicked up while you are moving bedding are not being inhaled by the horse.
- A nasal discharge is common first thing in the morning. If it is clear and odourless no action is needed; if the discharge is thick, cream, green, or foul-smelling, wipe it away and monitor how frequently this needs doing. If this continues for more than two days, or your horse's appetite decreases, call your vet, as secondary infections can develop if the airways are already inflamed.

WHAT YOUR VET MAY DO

If the horse is audibly wheezing – depending on the degree of difficulty your horse is having breathing – your vet may inject a drug that helps to relax the airways: bromhexine – otherwise known as ventipulmin – is currently the most used in the UK. They may also prescribe an oral form of the same drug which is mixed in the horse's food every day for long-term control and relief from symptoms. If there is any suspicion of a secondary infection your horse may also be prescribed antibiotics.

A persistent cough is most likely to be a combination of allergic airways and secondary bacterial infection taking advantage of the inflammation already present. Initially your vet will probably prescribe antibiotics; if these do not improve the condition, a more detailed investigation with an endoscope may be carried out. This may also include a **tracheal wash** or a **broncho-alveolar lavage**, which produces samples, taken directly from the upper airways, to look at cells and bacteria present. This allows your vet to tailor the treatment more exactly to your horse's condition.

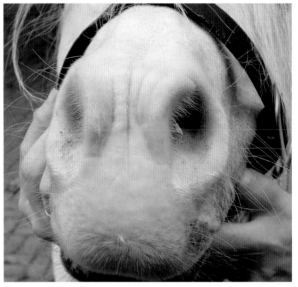

Flared nostrils when breathing at rest is a sign of airway disease and should be investigated

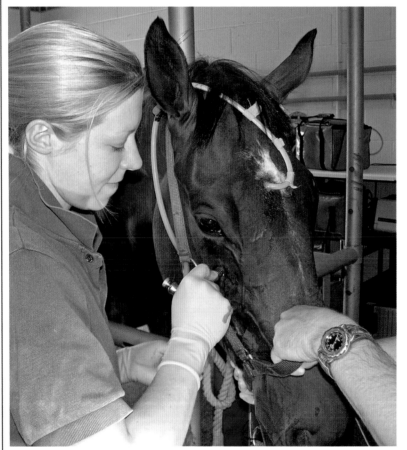

This horse has had two holes drilled into its skull: the upper one is clearly visible with tubing running into it, the lower one is just by the vet's hand. This combination will be used to flush saline or antibiotic-treated fluids through the sinus to clear a stubborn infection

If there is a nasal discharge, samples may be taken for examination and bacterial culture; the mouth may also be examined to check that there are no dental problems. Antibiotics may be prescribed once the type of infection has been identified.

WHAT CAN GO WRONG?

Repeated or poorly controlled episodes of airway inflammation can lead to permanent damage to the lung tissue, decreasing the elasticity of the airways and reducing lung capacity. Reduced lung capacity will in turn compromise the ability of the horse to exercise, and so also its performance potential.

FIRST AID FACTS

Nasal discharges and nosebleeds are a symptom of disease or injury within either the nasal cavity or the sinuses. Nasal discharge may simply be a 'head cold', or it may be a sinus infection, or a tooth root abscess.

The presence of tooth roots in the sinuses can mean that a tooth root abscess may initially show as a purulent nasal discharge. Here the pus will break out from the tooth root into the sinus and then drain down the nose.

NASAL DISCHARGE

WHAT TO LOOK FOR

- Most horses will have some discharge first thing in the morning, but as long as it is clear and runny there is nothing to worry about.
- If, however, the discharge is discoloured (creamy, pale yellow or green) or has a foul odour, there may be infection present.
- Check for spots of blood in the nasal discharge: this indicates very severe inflammation.

WHAT TO DO

- If your horse is otherwise bright and well in itself, wipe the discharge away regularly and it will probably clear up within two to three days.
- If your horse is off its food, seems dull or depressed, or there is a foul smell associated with the discharge, call your vet.

WHAT YOUR VET MAY DO

Nasal discharge is usually treated with antibiotics once the source of the infection has been found: this will involve checking the condition of the molars in case dental work is needed, or endoscopy to locate the root of the infection.

If the discharge proves stubborn to clear up, a period of time without antibiotics will be needed, and then a swab should be taken to try and identify the bacteria involved and a more accurately targeted antibiotic used.

Serious sinus infections may require more intensive treatment, for example a hole drilled into the side of the skull (trephination) to allow the use of sterile saline or antibiotic washes to flush out the infection more quickly.

WHAT CAN GO WRONG?

Deep-seated infections can be difficult to resolve, and extended courses of antibiotics may be required.

Nasal discharge may be related to guttural pouch mycosis, which can lead to damage to major blood vessels which run through this cavity (see Nosebleeds, page 50).

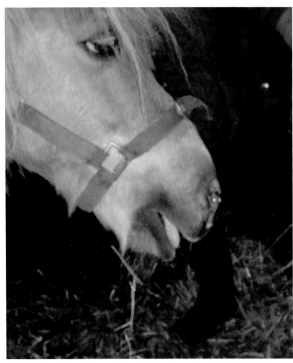

A thick mucous discharge combined with heavy breathing indicates a severe upper respiratory tract infection

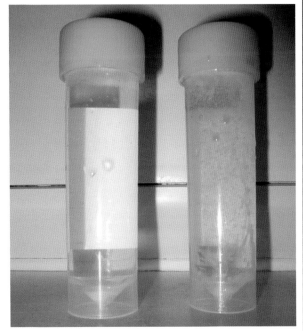

On the left is a normal sample taken from the trachea of a healthy horse – the fluid is almost clear; on the right is a cloudier, slightly bloody sample taken from the trachea of a horse with chronic airway inflammation

EQUINE 'FLU AND COLDS

FIRST AID FACTS

The equine influenza virus has a number of different strains named after the area and date of the epidemic associated with each one – for example Newmarket 1993 or Kentucky 1998.

Vaccination needs to be repeated annually in order to maintain protection against the virus. Most recognized equine organizations require evidence of vaccination against 'flu from horses participating at their events. The FEI is stricter and requires horses competing within its riules to have six-monthly 'flu boosters.

Other respiratory viruses include equine herpes virus, which most brood mares are vaccinated against, and equine viral arteritis.

WHAT TO LOOK FOR

- There will be a nasal discharge which initially will be clear and runny, but which often becomes yellow or green as secondary infections develop.
- Some horses develop a dry cough, initially only at exercise but gradually developing to coughing in the field or stable.
- General lethargy and lack of appetite: not being 'right'.
- Running a temperature.
- Check the glands at the angle of the jaw; if these are swollen it suggests that this may be strangles instead.

WHAT TO DO

- If you suspect 'flu, then you should isolate your horse as far as possible from all other horses, particularly any that have not been vaccinated.
- If your horse's appetite is reduced, offer small, frequent, palatable meals to encourage him to eat.

WHAT YOUR VET MAY DO

Following a full physical examination some swabs may be taken from the nose to determine which bacteria, if any, are involved, and in some cases to try to isolate the virus to confirm the diagnosis. Blood samples may also be taken to check organ function and the balance of red and white blood cells in the body. Antibiotics may be given to treat any secondary bacterial infections that may occur, and anti-inflammatories can be given to ease inflammation in the airways.

If your horse does not respond to treatment as expected, or the vet suspects there may be another underlying problem, then endoscopic examination of the airways may be carried out.

Once the illness has been controlled and your horse is fully recovered, your vet may discuss the use of improved vaccination or bio-security to prevent further problems in the future.

> **TOP TIP**
>
> Respiratory viral infections (colds) are more common in younger and older animals, because they have a slightly more vulnerable immune system.

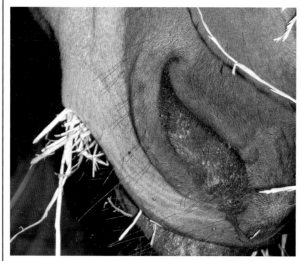

A small amount of discharge such as is shown here is normal to find in the nostril of a stabled horse

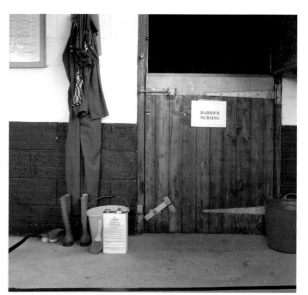

This picture illustrates the important factors in barrier nursing: it is clearly marked on the door, there is protective clothing, disinfectant, individual head collar and rope, grooming kit and skipping out bucket, and a clearly marked exclusion area on the floor. The infectious horse is on the end of the row so there is minimal passing foot traffic

WHAT CAN GO WRONG?

Chronic **viraemia** (low levels of virus remaining in the body) can be debilitating, and can have a similar effect to post-viral fatigue in humans. Affected horses need to be turned away to recuperate, which can take a few months. While the horse is turned away it will normally be given a vitamin and mineral supplement, and have monthly blood tests until a normal haematological picture returns (the balance of red and white cells returns to normal).

STRANGLES

FIRST AID FACTS

Strangles is caused by the bacteria *Streptococcus equi*, which is normally contracted in a similar way to colds. The bacteria is trapped in the lymph nodes of the neck (submandibular lymph nodes) where they start to divide rapidly, forming abscesses.

The infection can be transmitted on clothes, tack, buckets and in aerosol form; affected yards will be placed in quarantine until it has cleared up. It can be a debilitating condition but is rarely fatal, and once contracted, a degree of immunity to that strain of the bacteria will be developed. Younger horses are more susceptible to infection.

In rare cases the serious condition known as bastard strangles may develop: this is when the infection does not settle in the submandibular lymph nodes, but spreads into other lymph nodes in the chest and abdomen, causing internal abscesses.

WHAT TO LOOK FOR

- A high temperature.
- Not eating properly and general lethargy.
- A snotty nose, and swollen glands just behind the jaw.
- These swollen glands later progress to abscesses, which can then burst; there may also be a cough.

WHAT TO DO

- If you suspect strangles, then call your vet immediately and place your horse in quarantine. This means that it should be kept away from other horses, and you should not handle other horses, either.
- If your horse has lost its appetite, try feeding small, highly palatable meals frequently, making sure not to leave stale food in the stable as this can diminish appetite further.

WHAT YOUR VET MAY DO

Your horse will be isolated immediately, both from horses on the same yard and from those on surrounding grazing. A swab will be taken from the discharge in the nose to confirm that *Strep. equi* is present. Treatment will vary according to the stage of the infection.

If a horse on the same or a neighbouring yard is diagnosed with strangles but yours is not, it may be suggested that your horse is either treated with prophylactic antibiotics, or vaccinated against the disease.

WHAT CAN GO WRONG?

Strangles is an extremely infectious disease that will spread through an entire yard very quickly. The full-blown infection can be very debilitating, and it may take many months for your horse to recover full fitness and health.

In rare cases the abscesses can spread to other lymph nodes in the body, and if these burst it can prove fatal.

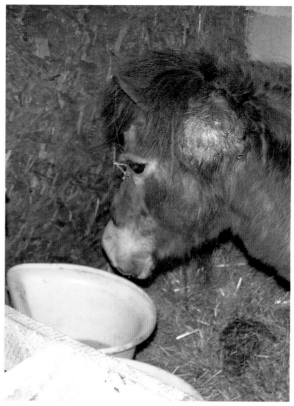

This pony has a large abscess typical of strangles

DIGESTION

THE BARE FACTS

Horses have a single simple stomach, similar in shape to a human's. It is physically impossible for a horse to be sick because of the strong cardiac sphincter ring of muscle joining the oesophagus to the stomach.

From mouth to tail the average horse's gut measures approximately 12m (40ft). The caecum is a blind-ended bag where bacteria ferment the fibrous food such as hay and grass to release the nutrition, which can then be absorbed and used by the body.

Signs of a healthy digestive system

- Healthy, stable appetite.
- Body condition is maintained easily.
- Sweet-smelling droppings are formed, with no mucus or blood.

Conditions affecting the digestion

- Colic.
- Diarrhoea.
- Choke.
- Poisoning.
- Dental disease.
- Tongue and gum problems.

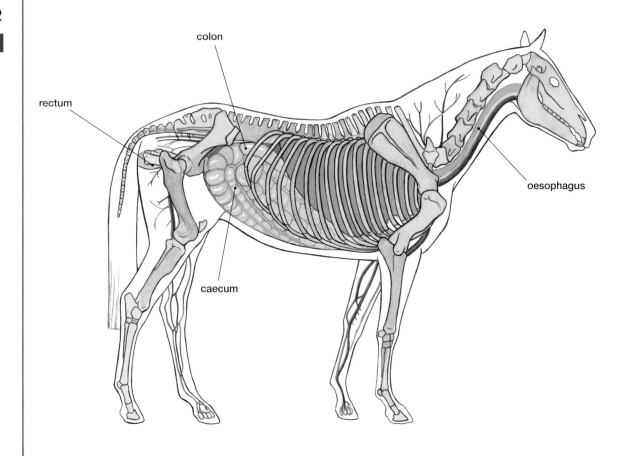

COLIC

FIRST AID FACTS

The horse's gut is a carefully balanced ecosystem of specialized bacteria which break down the high fibre content of the diet and release the nutrition for the horse to absorb. If the diet is changed suddenly the bacteria found in the gut will find it difficult to adapt, and this leads to either diarrhoea or a form of indigestion (colic).

Colic describes any form of abdominal pain, including pain caused by the other major organs such as liver, kidneys and the reproductive tract. Colic may be grouped into two major types:

- *Medical colic* caused by diarrhoea, gassy bloat, cramping guts (spasmodic colic), impaction or other abdominal pain.
- *Surgical colic* caused by twisted, trapped intestines.

An impaction is a form of constipation: the hindgut does a very sharp U-turn at the pelvis and narrows at the same time (**pelvic flexure**), and impactions commonly form here if the horse is not getting enough water, is not chewing well enough, or has a condition which is slowing down the movement of the gut (for example grass sickness). This form of colic, while being stubborn to respond to medical treatment, rarely progresses to require surgical treatment.

> **TOP TIP**
>
> Colic surgery is a very risky procedure with a poor recovery rate. It should only be considered in healthy horses that have been showing signs of colic for a short period of time and after serious discussion with your vet.

WHAT TO LOOK FOR

- Restlessness – rolling, kicking, sweating up.
- Not eating their normal food, or not drinking.
- Straining to pass faeces.
- Lying down for prolonged periods, often flat out.
- Rapid breathing, even when standing still.
- A change in the colour of the gums from salmon pink to grey or purple.

WHAT TO DO

- If you suspect colic, call your vet immediately.

WHAT YOUR VET MAY DO

The initial assessment will involve the vet listening to the heart rate, respiration rate and gut sounds, and looking at the colour of the gums to determine the severity of pain and the type of colic. If the colic is only mild, a drug will

---

'Old Wives' Tales'

'MYTH':
My horse has colic, can I walk it off?

VET'S REPLY:
This depends on the cause and severity of the colic symptoms: colic which is caused by too much gas, cramps in the guts, constipation or impaction can all be helped by movement – stubborn impactions are usually treated by a combination of laxatives and lungeing to encourage the gut to move normally again. Walking a horse with mild colic can distract the horse from its pain and help it relax, which in turn can help ease gut spasms; however, if a horse has severe colic symptoms and is continually trying to lie down and/or roll, then you must be very careful of both your own and your horse's safety. A colic that is caused by a twist in the gut will not be helped by movement – so always get your vet's advice before you walk your horse.

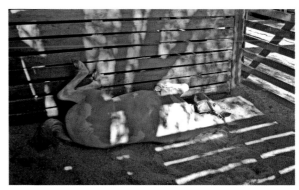

Rolling repeatedly is a symptom of colic

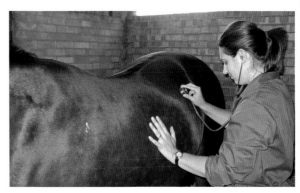

Listening to the gut sounds gives your vet clues about the cause of your horse's colic; lots of noise suggests a spasmodic colic, no gut sounds can indicate lack of movement in the guts, which is more serious

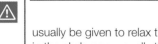

usually be given to relax the cramps and relieve the pain in the abdomen; usually this is enough to make the horse feel like eating again.

If the colic is more severe or the horse does not respond to medication, then a rectal examination may be carried out to assess the size and position of the guts. If there is a twist in the guts then the vet is usually able to identify large swollen loops of gut, which feel like bicycle tyres.

A stomach tube can be passed through the nostril, down the oesophagus into the stomach. If the guts are twisted close to the stomach, then the stomach will be full of fluid which can be drained out through the stomach tube; this gives temporary relief. A large volume of fluid being drained from the stomach gives a very poor prognosis because this means that a twist has been in place a long time in order for so much fluid to accumulate. If there is no fluid drained out through the stomach tube, or if the vet has felt an impaction during the rectal examination, then fluids and a laxative can be given via the tube.

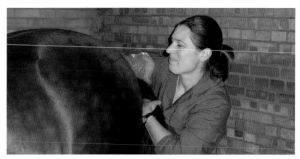

Rectal examination can be an important part of a colic examination, allowing the vet to tell if there is an impaction or a twist in the gut

To help clarify the exact nature of the problem in difficult cases a sterile needle may be put through the skin of the abdomen (peritoneal tap) to collect more information about the condition of the guts. The colour, type and volume of fluid will help to build a picture of the condition of the intestines.

Some referral centres are now using ultrasound examination to develop a clearer picture of what is happening in the abdomen of a horse with colic, although this is not yet routine.

Depending on the findings of these examinations, the horse can either be treated with drugs and/or laxatives, referred for surgery, or euthanased.

TOP TIP

Rectal examination in the horse can be risky as the gut lining is fragile and can tear. If you think your horse may object strongly to this type of examination, let your vet know so that a short-acting sedative can be given to make the examination safer for everyone involved.

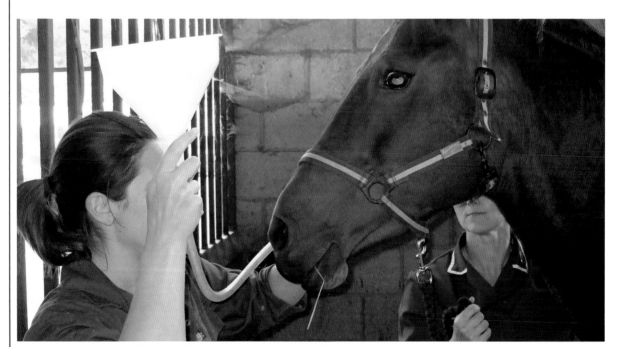

If a colic has been caused by impaction, or if your horse has choke, a stomach tube is passed via the nose, and fluids flushed into the stomach

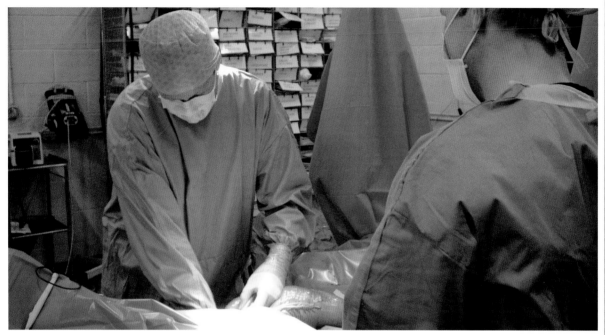

Colic surgery is a major undertaking: the risks involved in the anaesthetic, surgery and recovery are high, and it should not be undertaken lightly

WHAT CAN GO WRONG

Colic that requires surgery is an acute emergency: usually the horse is in very severe pain due to the loss of blood supply to a portion of the gut (known as *strangulation*). This can be caused either by the gut twisting on itself, or by a **pedunculated lipoma**: this is a small, benign fatty tumour on a stalk that wraps itself around a portion of gut like an overtight belt – this is a common cause of fatal colic in older horses.

Once the blood supply has been cut off, the gut dies and releases toxins that are absorbed through the **peritoneum**, the lining of the abdomen; these toxins can kill the horse even if the affected gut is removed, because they stay in the body and destabilize the cardiovascular

system: this is why speed is vital to the success of surgery should it be undertaken.

A heavy worm burden can cause colic through simple obstruction due to the volume of worms in the gut, or because the migrating worms damage the blood supply to the gut wall, causing **infarctions** (tissue death due to lack of blood supply). This is why it is very important to maintain a thorough and varied worming regime, and to keep pastures as clean as possible.

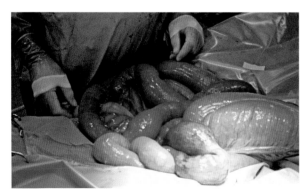

When the gut has been twisted, causing the colic, the surgeon must carefully lift it from the abdomen to assess the damage done, and attempt to correct it

65

'Old Wives' Tales'

'MYTH':
Drinking cold water after exercise causes colic.

VET'S REPLY:
During and immediately after exercise more blood is directed to the muscles than to the digestive tract; this means that drinking a large volume of cold water can cause pain in the stomach because the cold water causes the small blood vessels in the stomach lining to close up. A sudden reduction in blood supply causes cramps and severe pain, leading to colic symptoms – you will notice the same thing if you drink a large cold drink – but the pain eases as the fluid reaches body temperature and the blood vessels relax. Following intensive exercise the most effective method of rehydration is a body temperature electrolyte solution that the body will find easy to absorb quickly.

DIARRHOEA

FIRST AID FACTS

The greatest risk to the horse's health from diarrhoea is dehydration, because in severe cases it can be difficult for a horse or pony to drink as much fluid as it is losing in diarrhoea.

Antibiotics are rarely needed to treat diarrhoea, nor are they able to do so successfully, since it is most commonly caused by a sudden change of diet which disturbs the balance of bacteria in the hindgut, and causes inflammation of the gut lining, rather than being a consequence of infection.

Salmonellosis is a rare cause of diarrhoea but when it does occur it can make a horse gravely ill. Affected horses require intravenous fluid support, as loss of fluid due to diarrhoea can be so rapid that the horse is unable to replace it by drinking alone.

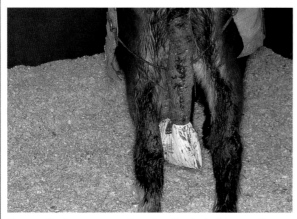

Severe diarrhoea causes faecal matter to build up on the tail and back legs; this in turn can 'scald' the skin and cause complications

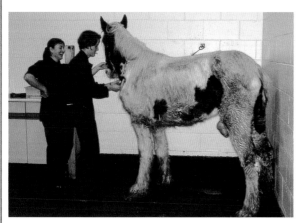

This horse has severe diarrhoea as a result of a high level of worms in the gut damaging the gut lining and interfering with digestion

WHAT TO LOOK FOR
- Loose or liquid droppings.
- The legs, haunches and tail will be covered with dried or wet faeces.
- There may be splatter marks from faeces up the walls of the stable.

> **TOP TIP**
>
> In rare cases *Salmonella* sp. and *E. coli* sp. can cause equine diarrhoea, so take very specific care of your personal hygiene.

WHAT TO DO
- Always change the diet gradually, as this allows the type of bacteria in the gut to adjust slowly so as to be able to digest the new diet.
- Remove all hard feed from your horse and restrict lush grazing, though ensure it has access to plenty of clean, fresh water.
- Encourage your horse to eat high fibre food such as hay or haylage.
- If the diarrhoea does not resolve or improve within two days, or if you suspect your horse is becoming dehydrated, call your vet.
- Keep any affected horses in quarantine to prevent the condition spreading through the yard.
- Keep your horse's tail and legs as clean as possible, because if faeces are left to dry on the skin for prolonged periods, the skin can scald.

> **TOP TIP**
>
> A cut-off leg from a pair of tights held in place by a tail bandage can keep the tail and dock as clean as possible, and is easy to wash and replace.

WHAT YOUR VET MAY DO

Most cases of diarrhoea can be dealt with without veterinary involvement, as mild cases may be treated simply with careful manipulation of the diet.

Severe cases that have not responded to a change to a high fibre diet, or where the diarrhoea is profuse, may require drugs to slow the movement of the gut and soothe the lining of the intestinal tract; these are administered either by stomach tube or by injection. If your horse is dehydrated, or at risk of becoming dehydrated, a drip may be placed to give intravenous fluid support; this replaces lost fluid, and also electrolytes. This is very important, as dehydration and an imbalance of electrolytes can rapidly become fatal if untreated.

Stubborn or recurrent cases may require a full medical work-up; this can include taking blood samples, faecal samples (to check for parasites and overgrowth of bacteria) or biopsies of the gut, and conducting a dental examination in order to pin-point the exact cause and to target effective treatment.

WHAT CAN GO WRONG?

If mild diarrhoea persists over a prolonged period and if there is significant faecal soiling of the hind limbs which is not cleaned away regularly, the skin can be literally burnt or scalded by the faecal material, leading to hair loss and ulceration, a condition which in itself may require veterinary treatment.

Untreated diarrhoea which persists or is severe can lead rapidly to dehydration, and to an imbalance in the electrolytes that are important in passing nerve messages and regulating cardiac function, both of which can kill a horse.

A heavy worm burden can cause diarrhoea by damaging the lining of the gut so that it is unable to absorb nutrients properly, which upsets the balance of the bacteria in the gut. This is why it is essential to maintain a regular worming programme.

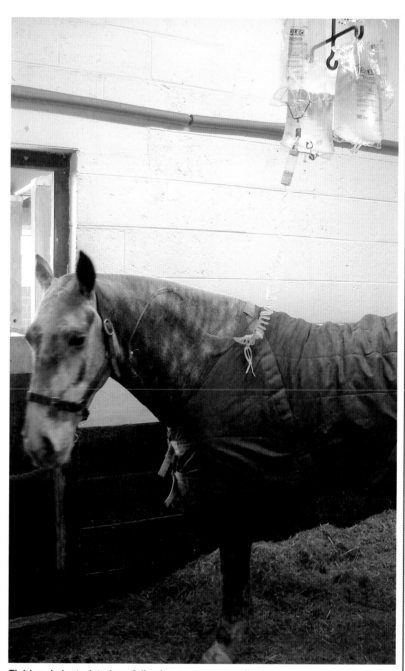

Fluid and electrolyte loss following acute severe diarrhoea can cause serious metabolic disturbances and should be rapidly corrected using aggressive intravenous fluid therapy

CHOKE

FIRST AID FACTS

Choke is the term used when a horse seems to have, or has, a blockage in its oesophagus (food pipe). This is normally caused by either swallowing a carrot, apple or similar which has not been properly chewed so it is too large to easily pass along the oesophagus into the stomach – typically the point of obstruction is at the point where the oesophagus passes from the neck into the chest (thoracic inlet). Greedy horses (or ponies) can also give themselves choke if they try to eat their concentrates too quickly and without chewing properly; this means that the food being swallowed is too dry and so sticks in the throat.

It is important that the type of feed should also be adjusted to suit the horse's personality: for example, a greedy horse will need to have its dry feed soaked thoroughly to prevent choke or swelling of the stomach, which can happen if dry food is eaten too quickly and does not soak up digestive juices until it is in the gullet or stomach.

WHAT TO LOOK FOR

- Suddenly stopping eating and looking worried in mid-feed.
- Wanting to drink or eat, but then shying away at the last minute.
- Food and saliva coming down both nostrils at once.
- A lump or swelling in the neck.
- The horse stretching out his neck and becoming increasingly distressed.

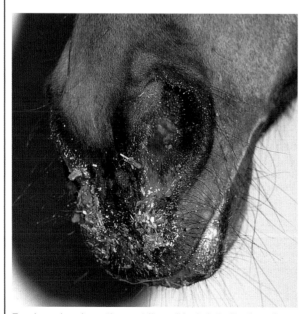

Food coming down the nostrils suddenly is indicative of choke

TOP TIP

Choke usually clears itself within twenty minutes if the horse is kept calm and away from further food.

WHAT TO DO

- Do not allow your horse to have access to food or water until the choke has cleared.
- If you can see a lump in the neck you can *gently* massage it to help loosen it.
- Choking can cause the horse to panic, especially if saliva comes down the nostrils, so try to keep your horse distracted, for example by grooming.
- If it does not clear or your horse is very distressed, call your vet.

WHAT YOUR VET MAY DO

A mild sedative or/and muscle relaxant can be given, which often allows the blockage to clear without further intervention. If this is not sufficient, then a stomach tube will be passed into the oesophagus via the nostril, and warm water flushed in repeatedly to loosen the obstruction and either flush it out or push it into the stomach; however, this can be a long and very messy procedure.

Once the obstruction is cleared, more warm water and electrolytes may be flushed into the stomach to replace the fluids lost while the horse was unable to swallow. Antibiotics and pain relief may be prescribed, depending on the severity of the choke and the damaged caused.

Very careful feeding will be required immediately afterwards as your horse will find swallowing quite uncomfortable; this usually means grass and water only, but your vet will discuss this in more detail once treatment is complete.

In very rare cases, if the obstruction does not move, then your horse may be referred for surgery.

WHAT CAN GO WRONG?

When the blockage has been difficult to clear there may be significant swelling of the oesophagus, which can make it painful and difficult for the horse to eat. This will increase the risk of the choke returning again (due to the narrowing of the gullet), and also of colic.

If choke is left untreated then the oesophagus may swell, increasing the pressure between the trapped food and the lining, which can lead to ulceration and secondary infection leading to serious complications.

If regurgitation occurs (that is, food coming down the nostrils), then there is a serious risk that the horse may inhale food particles, which can lead to the development of an aspiration pneumonia; this will require intensive antibiotic treatment.

POISONING

FIRST AID FACTS

Poisoning in horses is rare, as generally they are very careful about what they eat unless they are extremely hungry and there is nothing else to eat, especially as most toxic plants are quite bitter and unpalatable. Some plants are more toxic when they are dry than when they are fresh – for example, ragwort and St John's Wort; both of these plants can occasionally be found in poor quality hay.

WHAT PLANTS TO LOOK FOR

There are many other plants that are poisonous, and any plant in the paddock which is unfamiliar should be pulled up and identified.

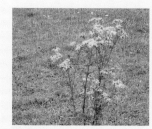

Ragwort

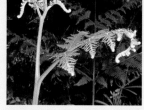

Bracken

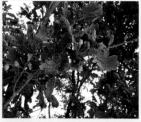

Acorns

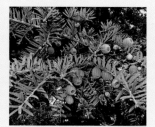

Yew

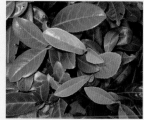

Laurel

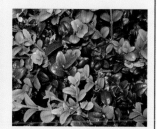

Box

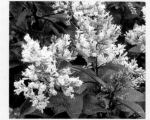

Privet

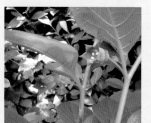

Nightshade plants

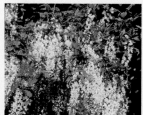

Laburnum

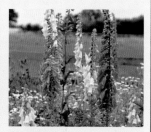

Foxgloves

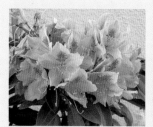

Rhododendrons

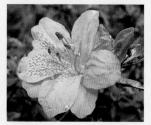

Azaleas

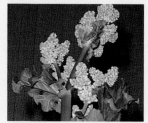

Rhubarb

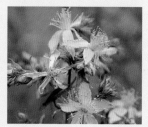

St John's Wort

69

WHAT TO LOOK FOR

- Poisoning in horses is not very common, and symptoms will vary depending on the toxin involved; anything consistently abnormal should be investigated.
- Poisons which irritate the lining of the digestive tract will cause either colic symptoms or diarrhoea.
- Chronic poisoning will cause a gradual loss in condition and often mild recurrent colic symptoms.
- If you suspect poisoning, search the field closely for any plants which appear to have been grazed, check the hay for any rogue ragwort, and make sure that nothing has been fed to the horse as a titbit by well-meaning passers-by or neighbours.

WHAT TO DO

- If you suspect poisoning, call the vet immediately and then search for the possible source of a toxin.

WHAT YOUR VET MAY DO

Some poisons have specific treatments, so if you have any suspicions about the cause, tell the vet so that accurate treatment can be started immediately.

Where poisoning is suspected but not confirmed, treatment will be symptomatic – that is, aimed at relieving the symptoms as they arise while carrying out tests to pinpoint the cause. Many poisons are *ingested* so treatment is initially directed towards protecting the gut and stopping further absorption of toxins.

Supportive treatment often involves intravenous fluids to help dilute and flush the toxins out of the body, while oral treatments can be given to protect the gut lining from the abrasive effects of the poisons and prevent anything further being absorbed into the body.

GRAIN (CARBOHYDRATE) OVERLOAD

If your horse breaks into the feed bin or grain store and gorges itself (this can be on wheat, oats or barley), it can cause catastrophic changes in the digestive system. The fermentation of the grain will kill all the friendly bacteria that the horse needs for digestion, and will cause serious diarrhoea and serious sudden-onset laminitis. In many cases this is fatal. If you suspect your horse has gorged itself in this way, call the vet immediately: laxatives can be given to move the grain through the gut faster, and special absorbents can also be given which soak up the toxins produced by the fermentation of the grain.

WHAT CAN GO WRONG?

Some poisoning can cause irreparable damage to organs, which ultimately results in the horse needing to be euthanased. Grain overload can cause such severe changes in the digestive system and subsequent laminitis that successful treatment is not possible, and this will also result in euthanasia.

RAGWORT POISONING

Ragwort poisoning often happens over a prolonged period of time, usually from eating small amounts of ragwort in the hay or at pasture over a number of seasons. Clinical symptoms only become apparent when the liver is sufficiently scarred (*cirrhosed*) to be unable to recover, so treatment can only be supportive, and cannot be curative.

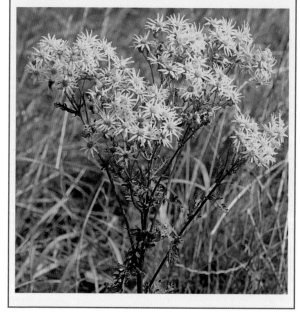

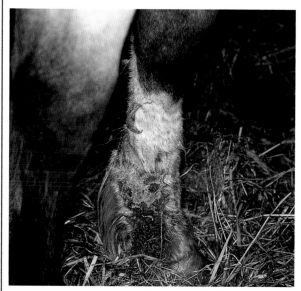

The white area on the fetlock of this horse is ulcerated and inflamed as a result of liver failure caused by ragwort poisoning. This is known as photosensitivity

DENTAL DISEASE

FIRST AID FACTS

Dental disease in horses is extremely common. It can be caused by a number of factors, including dietary problems, genetic predisposition and old age.

The adult teeth grow constantly throughout the horse's life, and change shape as they erupt; they are designed to be gradually worn down by chewing grass and hay.

A concentrate diet does not wear the teeth adequately, and also changes the pattern of chewing – this can lead to an overgrowth of parts of the tooth, causing pain, and further affecting the range of chewing.

The horse has between 42 and 46 adult teeth (depending on the presence of wolf teeth and tushes). There is an extensive system of air-filled sinuses in the head to keep the skull a relatively light weight for its size. The upper molar roots extend into the sinus cavity, and infection in the roots of one of these teeth will cause a foul nasal discharge.

A horse's teeth should be checked regularly, at least once a year, and any problems dealt with on a routine basis. Dental treatment should be performed by either a vet or a qualified dental technician.

WHAT TO LOOK FOR

- To check for a healthy mouth, hold your horse's nose in one hand and the lower jaw in the other: you should be able to move the lower jaw sideways in both directions at least the distance of the width of one incisor. Now stand to the side of your horse and lift the head up, and then tuck the chin down and in: you should see the lower incisors move slightly backwards as the head goes up, and slightly forwards as the head comes down, the teeth sliding over each other.

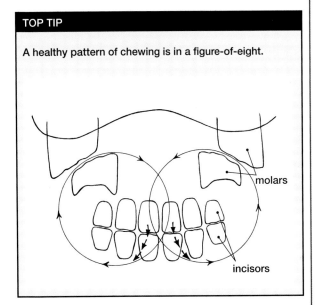

- Watch for **quidding**, when your horse is struggling to chew or swallow properly, so half-chewed food is dropped out of the mouth. This is easiest to spot under the haynet, as the horse is standing eating in one spot for an extended period of time.
- A swelling developing on the face – this can be either trapped food in the mouth or an abscess.
- If your horse is slowly losing weight.
- If there is a foul smell coming from the mouth.
- Sudden discomfort in the mouth, refusing to take the bit or reacting against the bit when being ridden.

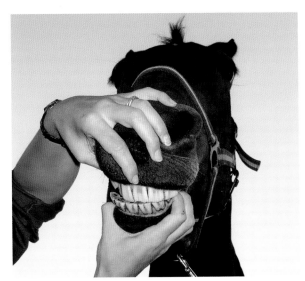

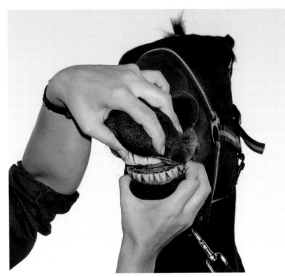

You should be able to slide your horse's mouth from side to side approximately one incisor-width, each way

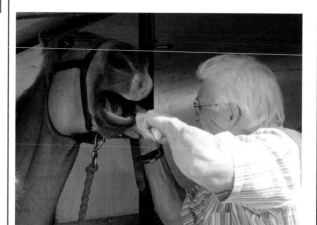

Regular dental treatment is important in order to maintain good oral health

TOP TIP

In young horses – generally at two to three years – the roots of the adult molars can be felt under the jaw bone: these are known as *juvenile bumps*.

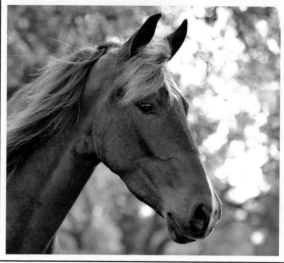

WHAT TO DO
- If you suspect your horse has dental pain, then soaking the food or turning the nuts into a soup will make it easier for the horse to continue eating, and so prevent loss of condition.
- You will need to speak to your vet and plan a full examination of the mouth; the vet will undoubtedly need to use a Hausman's gag.

WHAT YOUR VET OR DENTIST MAY DO
A thorough inspection of the mouth requires the use of a hausman gag. However, many horses do not tolerate this procedure very well and may require sedation to enable a full examination and effective treatment.

Once a problem is identified it can be corrected either by rasping (by hand, or with a motorized rasp) or by removing the tooth if it is cracked, loose or badly infected. Severely damaged or infected molars may need to be done under general anaesthetic. Antibiotics, antiseptic mouth washes and pain relief are often used to speed recovery.

There is often the need for repeated corrective work, as changing the balance of the mouth too quickly can cause further problems; and many problems are caused by poor conformation of the mouth, and as such will be ongoing.

72

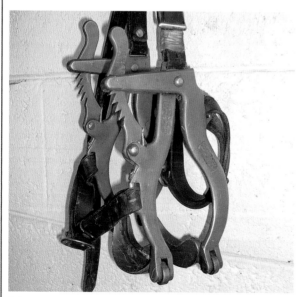

A hausman gag

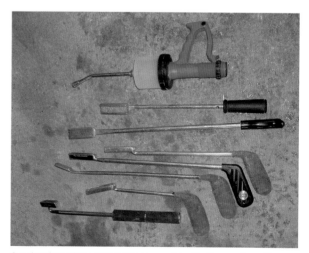

A selection of the hand rasps used to file the molars: the different angles of the heads allow good access to the difficult parts of the mouth

WHAT CAN GO WRONG?

Poor conformation of the mouth can lead to the formation of hooks (overgrowth of the front of the first upper molar) and ramps (overgrowth of the back of the last lower molar); these are generally caused by a malformation of the opposing tooth, so there is no opposing surface to wear against. These hooks and ramps can grow sufficiently large that they can rub against the opposite gums, causing ulceration, infection and pain.

A high sugar diet can lead to cavities in the same manner as in humans. Furthermore, feeding a diet that is low in fibre causes an abnormal chewing pattern so teeth do not wear properly, and sharp spurs develop that may cut into the tongue (lower molars) or cheek (upper molars): these are painful, and can become infected.

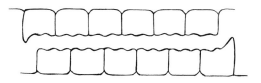

Hooks (above left) and ramps (above right) need to be dealt with by your equine dentist to create a correct chewing surface (below)

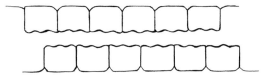

TONGUE AND GUM PROBLEMS

FIRST AID FACTS

The mouth heals very quickly, and usually even major wounds are almost healed within a week. If the tongue is painful, however, the horse will find swallowing difficult, will drool and be off its food.

Brambles, or other foreign bodies, can become embedded in the gums, lips or tongue and cause infection. Gingivitis is uncommon, and is usually only seen in relation to the build-up of plaque and tartar, for example on the **tushes**.

WHAT TO LOOK FOR

- Changes in eating habits; if your horse has mouth pain, then soft food is preferred to hay and nuts.
- Drooling and dropping food from the mouth.
- Spots of blood in the food or water bucket, or on food dropped from the mouth.
- Gingivitis: increased redness, caused by inflammation, particularly around the teeth.
- The tongue should be smooth and even in shape and texture; any blistering or redness is abnormal.

WHAT TO DO

- Call your vet, because the mouth will require close examination to determine the cause of the pain.
- Feed sloppy, wet food to allow your horse to eat with minimal discomfort until your vet can visit.

WHAT YOUR VET MAY DO

A full examination of the mouth usually requires a Hausman's gag to allow a clear view of the whole mouth. This will allow the vet to make a thorough check for any foreign bodies, and to locate the focus of the pain so that appropriate treatment can start.

Very few injuries in the mouth require suturing, unless it is a long laceration or goes through the cheek and penetrates the skin. Most tongue injuries will heal with careful dietary management, antibiotics and pain relief.

WHAT CAN GO WRONG?

Most mouth injuries heal very quickly and without any complications; however, injuries to the tongue may make your horse less tolerant of the bit.

Some gum conditions may require ongoing treatment; for instance, gingivitis can cause gum recession if it is untreated, which in turn can lead to a loosening of the teeth, and eventually their loss.

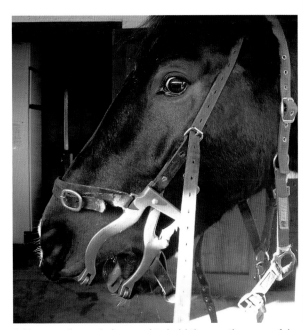

A Hausman's gag being used to hold the mouth open safely for full dental examination and treatment

THE UROGENITAL SYSTEM

THE BARE FACTS

The horse reaches puberty between 18 months and two years of age, but despite this a filly will not normally become pregnant until she is three or four years of age. The reproductive cycle of the mare is usually 21 to 24 days, although as with all species there is generally some individual variation.

Mares naturally come into season in the spring so that the foal produced the following year will be born when the grass is at its best.

The gestation period (length of pregnancy) of the horse is 11 months (330 to 345 days), although pregnancy can extend to a little over 365 days.

TOP TIP

Thoroughbred horses can only be registered if conceived by natural service.

Signs of a healthy urogenital tract

- No discharge from the tip of the penis or from the vulva.
- No sign of pain or straining when urinating.
- No sudden change in the volume of water drunk or the amount of urine produced.
- No swellings or sores around the genitalia.

TOP TIP

Horse urine has a higher mucus content than the urine of many other mammals, giving it a cloudy appearance which can appear abnormal.

Conditions affecting the urogenital tract

- Infection of the urinary tract
- Bladder stones
- Infection of the uterus
- Penile prolapse
- Inguinal hernia
- Mastitis

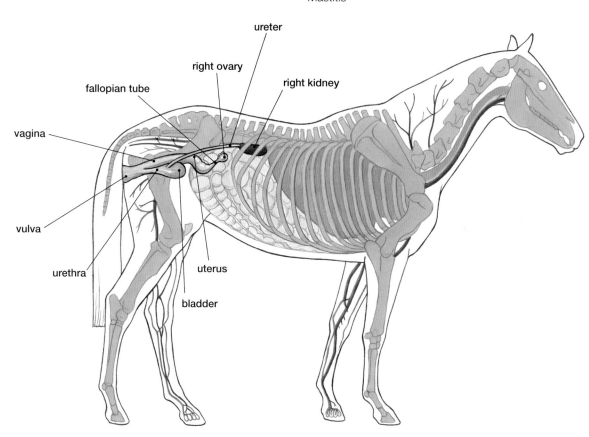

INFECTION OF THE URINARY TRACT

FIRST AID FACTS
Bacterial infection of the urinary tract is uncommon. Cystitis is seen more frequently in females than males, because the urethra is much shorter so bacteria have a short distance to travel to the bladder. In very rare cases infection can spread into the ureters and the kidneys: this condition is called pyelonephritis.

WHAT TO LOOK FOR
- Frequently passing small volumes of urine.
- Showing pain when passing urine.
- Blood in the urine.
- A change in the smell of the urine: it will become foul-smelling.
- A high temperature.
- A lack of appetite.
- Occasionally abdominal pain will be shown as colic.

WHAT TO DO
- Ensure an ample supply of fresh water at all times.
- Add water to normal feeds to increase water intake.
- Collect a sample of urine if possible; the easiest way to do this is to collect a sterile sample pot and some long gloves from your vets, and wait and watch.
- If you suspect an infection, call your vet for advice.

WHAT YOUR VET MAY DO
A urine sample will be needed to evaluate the number of red and white blood cells, and the bacteria present. This is usually collected mid-flow. A catheter may be placed into the bladder to collect a sample directly. A second sample may be taken into a special preservative for bacterial culture to identify the bacteria and the most effective antibiotics.

The vet may check your horse's temperature to determine whether the infection is localized, or if it has spread into the rest of the body. The external genitalia will be examined for any indication of the cause of the infection – for example, faecal contamination of the vagina, or a build-up of smegma in the foreskin.

The vet will also conduct a rectal examination to check that the size and shape of the bladder is normal, and for any other obvious abnormalities that may have predisposed the horse to an infection. A blood sample may be taken to identify if the infection is isolated in the bladder or has extended to the kidneys.

Treatment for a urinary tract infection will most likely include a prolonged course of antibiotics, pain relief may be given depending on the condition of the kidneys, and feed additives in order to adjust the pH of the urine to make conditions more difficult for the bacteria to continue multiplying.

WHAT CAN GO WRONG?
Infection that spreads to the kidneys can cause long-term damage to kidney function, or in extreme cases can lead to kidney failure.

Undetected chronic infection can cause the formation of bladder stones as a reaction to the presence of bacteria in the urine.

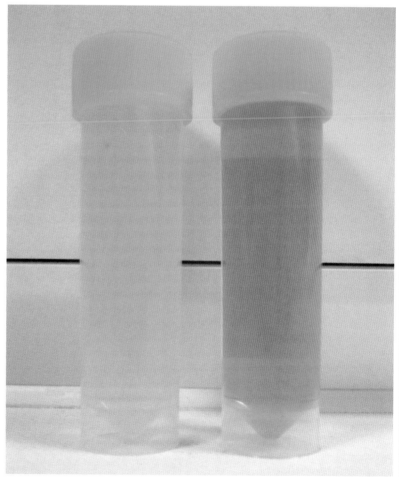

On the left is a normal urine sample: the cloudiness is due to the horse having more mucus in its urine than other mammals. The urine sample on the right has blood in it, which is indicative of disease in the urinary tract; severe cases may even have blood clots

BLADDER STONES

FIRST AID FACTS

Stones can form anywhere in the urinary tract, though the bladder is the most common site. Bladder stones can obstruct the urinary tract if they leave the bladder and become stuck in the urethra; this is more common in males as the urethra is longer with more bends.

WHAT TO LOOK FOR

- The presence of blood, blood clots, pus or other debris in the urine.
- Pain on passing urine.
- Colic symptoms.
- Inability to pass urine.

WHAT TO DO

- Ensure an ample supply of fresh water, unless you think your horse is unable to pass urine, in which case you must call your vet immediately.
- If possible collect a urine sample for analysis and see your vet for advice.

WHAT YOUR VET MAY DO

Your vet may perform a rectal examination to confirm if the bladder is full or empty: an empty bladder will allow confirmation of bladder stones as they can be felt through the bladder wall, whereas a full bladder – despite straining to pass urine – suggests that a stone has become stuck in the urethra.

A catheter can be passed into the urethra to take a sterile urine sample to check for the presence of crystals or small stones.

If a stone is stuck in the urethra a muscle relaxant may be given to relax the urethra, which may be sufficient to allow the stone to pass. In some cases, passing the catheter may move the stone back into the bladder. Surgery may be required to remove the stones from either the urethra or the bladder.

WHAT CAN GO WRONG?

In rare cases, obstruction of the urinary tract can lead to damage to the kidneys from the build-up of urine; and in very rare cases the bladder can rupture.

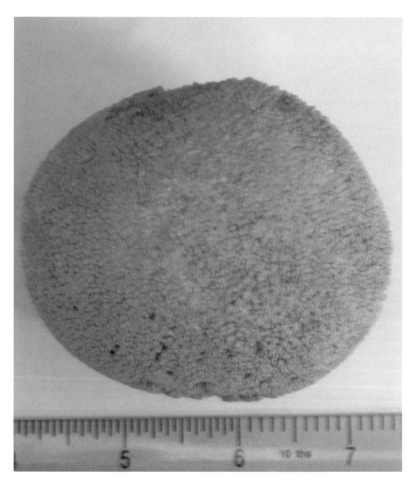

A bladder stone of this size will cause significant discomfort and often colic symptoms, it can only be safely removed surgically

INFECTION OF THE UTERUS

FIRST AID FACTS

The uterus has a very effective built-in immune system, which becomes more active during heats because this is the time when bacteria (from mating) are most likely to be introduced into the genital tract.

Infection of the uterus is called endometritis; in very severe cases where pus has built up in the uterus, this is termed pyometra. It is believed that poor conformation of the external reproductive tract is a significant factor in this condition.

WHAT TO LOOK FOR

- Any discharge coming from the vulva, particularly following a mating.
- A shorter than normal cycle, usually only 16 days rather than 21.

WHAT TO DO

- Prevention is more effective than treatment: if you are breeding from your mare, ensure that both the stallion's penis and her external genitalia are clean before service.
- If you suspect that infection is present, call your vet for advice.

WHAT YOUR VET MAY DO

Ultrasound examination of the reproductive tract per rectum will show any abnormal fluid in the uterus, which is suggestive of infection. Swabs may be taken to isolate the bacteria involved.

Initial treatment usually involves manipulation of the oestrus cycle to bring the mare into season to allow her own immune system to deal with infection. In some cases oxytocin may be used to stimulate contraction of the uterus to push out the contaminated material, or the uterus can be washed out with a sterile saline, or in some cases an antiseptic solution.

Once treatment is under way, the likely causative factors – these could be air or faecal material contaminating the vagina – will be identified and corrected.

WHAT CAN GO WRONG?

Chronic or recurrent infections of the uterus can result in permanent damage to the uterine lining, and this will cause infertility.

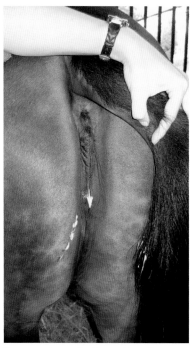

If you notice a discharge from the vulva it can indicate an infection of the vagina or uterus; veterinary advice should be sought

77

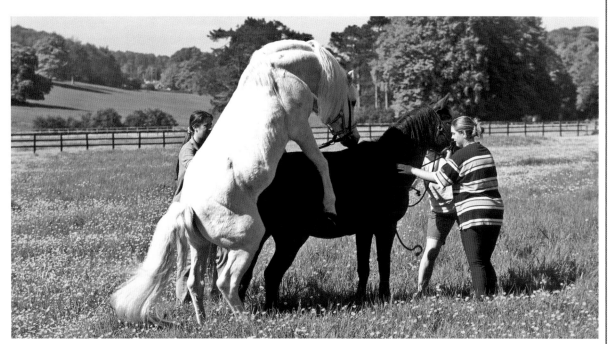

To maintain the good health of the uterus it is important to check the health state of the stallion before service

PENILE PROBLEMS

FIRST AID FACTS

The smegma produced by the horse is carcinogenic, and in rare cases can lead to the development of aggressive tumours on the surface of the penis. Smegma can build up under the foreskin, forming stones which are very painful, and can provoke colic symptoms.

Infection can develop in the sheath, which causes swelling and an abnormal gait; if it is very painful the horse may show colic symptoms.

A sedative used on horses (acepromazine – ACP) has the effect of relaxing the muscles controlling the penis, causing it to drop out fully without erection. This can be very useful for cleaning it if there are any associated problems.

WHAT TO LOOK FOR

- The penis should be a smooth, tubular organ of equal thickness along its length.
- The sheath should be soft and relaxed in appearance, with no discharge.
- Some peeling skin along the shaft is normal, but build-up of dead skin can cause irritation and inflammation.
- There should be no lumps along the length of the shaft.

WHAT TO DO

- Most male horses benefit from a routine cleaning of the penis: there are special cleaning agents available for this. This clean should be used to check for lumps, bumps and the build-up of material along the shaft.
- The frequency of this cleaning routine varies between different horses: if in doubt, discuss with your veterinary surgeon at a routine visit.

- If your horse has had a sedative, monitor the retraction of the penis: it should have returned to its normal position by the time the sedative has worn off. If it does not, call your vet for advice.

WHAT YOUR VET MAY DO

Any abnormalities in the shape of the penis should be investigated; biopsies may need to be taken to determine if further treatment – including surgical removal – is required. Sedation is likely to be used to drop the penis from the sheath and allow safe, close examination and treatment.

If your horse fails to retract its penis (paraphimosis) the first factor to be assessed is whether it can urinate. Depending on the cause of the condition, massage may be used to reduce the fluid build-up – though if the problem has been caused by bruising from an injury from breeding, this may not be advisable!

Supportive bandages can be made to measure to support the body of the penis and prevent further fluid build-up that would add weight and make the penis less likely to retract naturally. Lubrication will be required until the penis can be retracted.

WHAT CAN GO WRONG?

In severe cases, tumours or an otherwise badly damaged penile body may require amputation. This does not affect the ability of the horse to urinate, but in stallions it does mean the loss of mating ability.

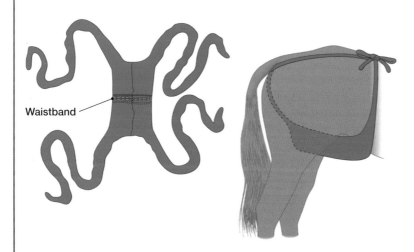

Waistband

Two pairs of tights sewn together at the waistband provide a long and wide supportive base for the penis, while the legs of the tights provide a flexible, supportive attachment

INGUINAL HERNIA

FIRST AID FACTS

The inguinal ring is a small triangular gap in the groin where the abdominal muscles meet. In males, this is the route that the testicles pass through when they descend from the abdomen into the scrotum, usually within two weeks of birth. This gap, although normally very small, opens directly into the abdomen.

Stallions, colts shortly after gelding, and newborn foals are at greatest risk of developing hernia (where the abdominal contents escape through the inguinal ring).

WHAT TO LOOK FOR

- A sudden swelling in the groin, usually associated with colic symptoms.
- In entire stallions, one testicle will suddenly be much larger than the other.

WHAT TO DO

- This is an emergency, because the blood supply to any tissue slipping through the inguinal ring may be cut off, so a vet must be called immediately.

WHAT YOUR VET MAY DO

In newborn foals usually no treatment is necessary as long as the hernia does not increase in size and there are no colic symptoms.

Ultrasound examination or rectal examination may be used to confirm and identify abdominal contents in the hernia. Emergency surgical treatment may be required under general anaesthetic to replace the gut contents into the abdomen and close the inguinal ring so the problem cannot recur.

WHAT CAN GO WRONG?

In the worse case scenario, gut can become trapped in the hernia and lose its blood supply and die off. This is extremely serious; it may be surgically correctable depending on the amount of gut involved, and whether blood poisoning and shock have developed.

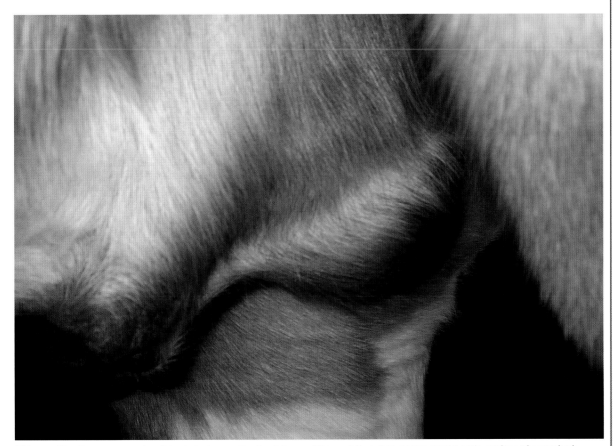

This swelling has appeared suddenly between the back legs of this gelding: it is an inguinal hernia and needs surgical correction

MASTITIS

FIRST AID FACTS
Mastitis is a bacterial infection of the mammary glands (udder), usually seen in lactating mares, although occasionally maiden mares can be affected.

WHAT TO LOOK FOR
- Heat and swelling in the udder; often one side is larger than the other.
- Walking with a stiff gait.
- Striking out, out of character, when you groom under the abdomen.
- Not allowing the foal to suckle.

WHAT TO DO
- If you think your mare has mastitis, call your vet for advice straightaway.
- If your mare has a foal, you may need to bottle feed it until the mare has recovered.

WHAT YOUR VET MAY DO
A sample of milk may be taken for examination if your mare is lactating. Antibiotics and pain relief are likely to be given; mastitis can be a stubborn condition, so a prolonged course of antibiotics may be required.

WHAT CAN GO WRONG?
If the infection is difficult to control or causes extensive damage the udder may be permanently damaged and unable to produce milk in the future.

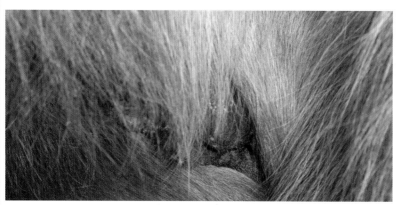

A normal udder

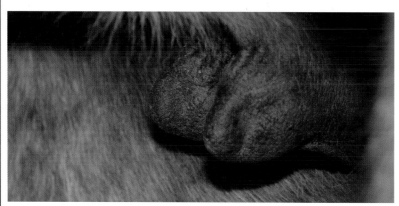

Swelling and tenderness of the udder suggests that an infection, known as mastitis, has developed

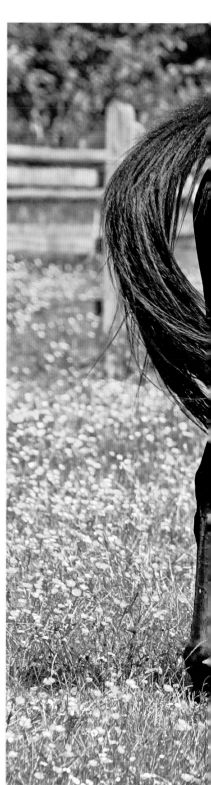

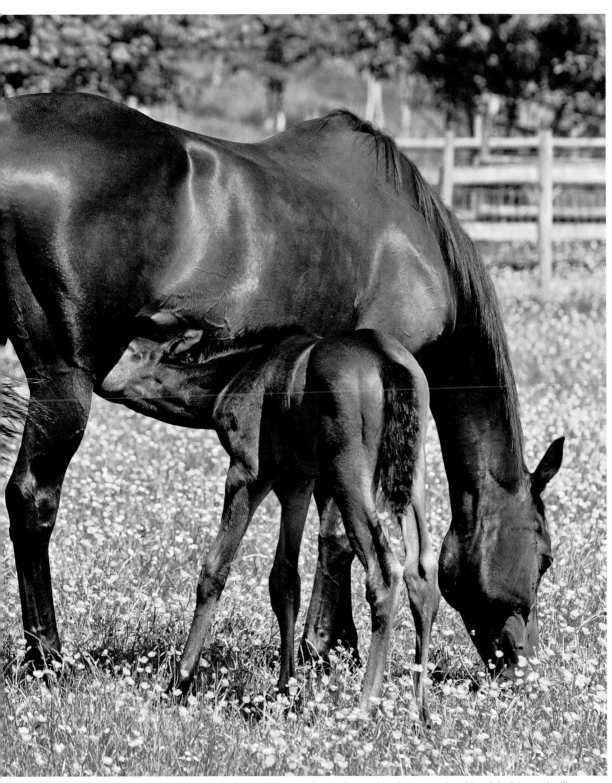

A foal with a good appetite will suckle regularly helping to maintain the health of the mare's udder. A build-up of milk caused by a weak foal not suckling properly is a pre-disposing factor for mastitis

MUSCLES AND TENDONS

THE BARE FACTS

There are two different types of muscle: smooth muscle, which is controlled without conscious thought, for example the gut; and striated muscle, which is involved in voluntary movement. Electrolytes, as well as calcium, are very important in the normal healthy function of muscles, which is why dehydration can have such serious knock-on effects.

Even though muscle and tendon injuries might appear to take precedence as a cause of lameness, 80–90 per cent of lameness in fact originates in the foot, not the leg.

Injuries to the soft tissues can take significant periods of time to heal completely; in the case of serious tendon damage, this can be up to 18 months.

Signs of healthy muscles and tendons
- Clean, smooth lines with no swelling.
- Smooth, easy action when moving.
- Symmetrical limbs and muscles.

Conditions affecting muscles and tendons
- Tying up (azoturia, or exertional rhabdomyolysis).
- Muscle or tendon strain, sprain or tear.
- A cast horse.
- Back pain (muscle spasm).

THE STAY APPARATUS

The stay apparatus is unique to the horse; it is a combination of tendons and ligaments that allows a horse to stand for long periods without the muscles becoming tired.

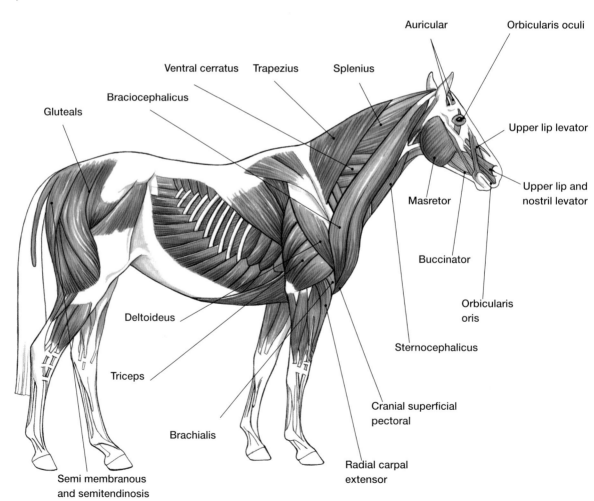

TYING UP

FIRST AID FACTS

Tying up, also known as azoturia, Monday morning sickness or, more correctly, exertional rhabdomyolysis, is caused by an imbalance of electrolytes in the body of the muscle resulting in a sensation equivalent to cramp. There is no definitive cause of this problem: it is usually seen in fit horses that work hard, have a day off, and then work hard again. It generally develops while at work, or shortly after the end of exercise.

Once a horse has suffered from azoturia it is prone to repeat attacks, and as a result changes may need to be made in the balance of nutrients in the diet, and in the way the horse is managed.

TOP TIP

Horses affected by azoturia require a diet low in carbohydrates and high in fibre with supplemented minerals and vitamins to minimize the risk of recurrence.

WHAT TO LOOK FOR

- During work the paces may become short, stiff and uneven, with the horse gradually becoming less willing to move.
- The muscles of the hindquarters will feel rock hard to the touch and may be extremely painful.
- Horses in a great deal of pain may lie down and refuse to move.
- If the horse is in a lot of pain it may not want to eat or drink, and without treatment may develop colic as a secondary problem.
- In severe cases the urine becomes red brown.

WHAT TO DO

- **DO NOT MAKE THE HORSE MOVE MORE THAN IS ABSOLUTELY NECESSARY AS THIS CAN CAUSE PERMANENT MUSCLE DAMAGE AND MAY ALSO LEAD TO KIDNEY FAILURE.**
- Dismount and lead your horse slowly to the stable. If this becomes difficult, or if you are a long way from home, arrange for a trailer to collect the horse and transport it home.
- Rug your horse up to maintain warmth, particularly if it is sweating as this can rapidly chill the muscles and cause further pain.
- Offer the horse plenty of fluids, either normal water or electrolytes, to help flush from its system the toxins produced by the cramping muscles.
- If your horse is not moving more freely within half an hour, phone your vet for advice.

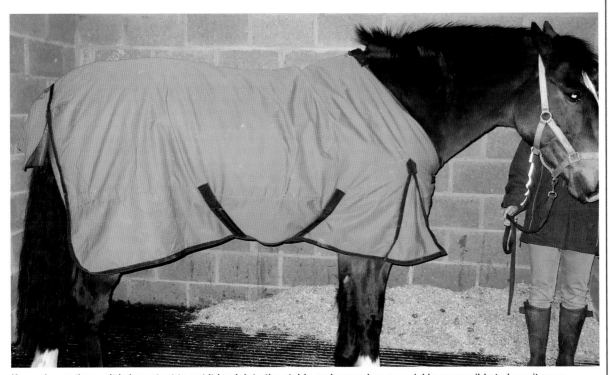

If your horse ties up it is important to get it back into the stable and rugged up as quickly as possible to keep it warm

WHAT YOUR VET MAY DO

The treatment given will depend on how badly the muscles are affected. Mild cases may improve with a combination of painkillers and a drug to improve the blood supply through the muscles, combined with strict rest and warmth.

More severe cases may also need intravenous fluids to flush from the body the toxins produced by the muscles in a dilute form to reduce the damage to the kidneys, and also to replace electrolytes so as to restore a normal balance in the blood and in the muscles.

The vet will advise you on changes to your training/ exercise regime and how to manipulate the diet to reduce the risk of recurrence.

WHAT CAN GO WRONG?

Horses that are repeatedly affected may be increasingly less able to tolerate exercise, and may become unsuitable for the purpose for which they are kept.

Severe cases can take a prolonged period to recover, and this may as a result leave the muscles scarred and prone to recurrent bouts of tying up.

In very severe cases, where there is extensive muscle damage and subsequent breakdown, the by-product (myoglobin) is removed from the body via the urinary tract. This produces a red or brown discoloration in the urine; at very high levels the myoglobin causes severe kidney damage which can develop into kidney failure.

TOP TIP

Advice regarding diet and nutrition following a bout of azoturia will vary between individual horses, depending on how severely affected the horse has been and what it is used for. This is an area which is the subject of much research by nutritionists, and advice is likely to change as understanding improves.

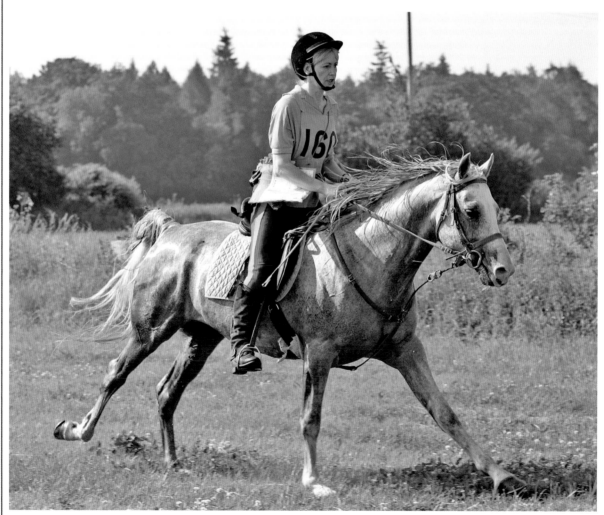

Endurance horses work at a very high level over a prolonged period which makes them prone to tying up following a competition

TENDON INJURIES

FIRST AID FACTS

Muscle and tendon injuries can occur in any horse at any level of fitness, either at work or in the field, but recuperation will almost always involve as little exercise as possible.

Muscles and tendons can be either strained or torn; strains heal more quickly and more easily. Inactivity is the best way to encourage healing, and this usually means box rest – although some horses may resent this and then have to be confined to a very small paddock (play pen) if they box walk.

A horse can function without the tendons that run down the front of the leg, but any injury that severs the tendons at the back of the leg is very serious and may not be treatable – classically when there is rupture of the flexor tendons the foot does not sit flat on the ground but the toe is lifted up, even at rest.

WHAT TO LOOK FOR

- **Muscle and tendon strains**: there is often sudden onset mild or severe lameness, with heat and swelling in the affected soft tissue. It usually occurs at exercise, but it can happen in the field during play.
- **Tendon tear**: there is sudden onset severe lameness, with rapid swelling of the affected lower limb (this is sometimes referred to as a **bowed tendon**).
- **Severed tendon**: if one or both of the major tendons running down the back of the leg is severed the foot will no longer sit flat on the ground but will have the toe pointing upwards.

> **TOP TIP**
>
> If your horse has arthritis or allergy problems you will need to discuss this with your vet, as this could affect how your horse is confined while the injury heals.

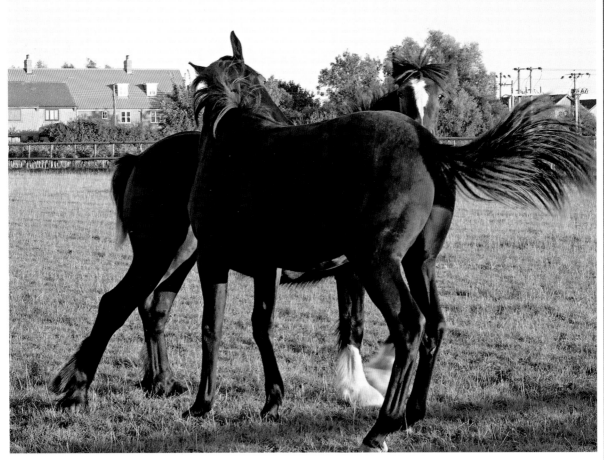

Youngsters playing in the field can get carried away and injure themselves

WHAT TO DO

- If you suspect soft tissue injury while riding, dismount immediately, walk your horse home, and apply cold water or cooling bandages to the affected areas.
- If you suspect a serious tendon injury you should call your vet immediately.
- If you think your horse has a strain, keep cooling the swollen area, then dry it carefully and put supportive stable bandages on all the legs, keep the horse in the stable overnight and reassess the situation in the morning. If the horse is still in pain, and/or the tendon swollen and painful to touch, call your vet for advice.

'Old Wives' Tales'

'MYTH':
Please don't give my horse any pain relief: it will move around too much and make an injury worse.

VET'S REPLY:
There are two different ways that pain relief works: the most common class of pain relief in horses are the non-steroidal anti-inflammatories (NSAIDs), being the same type of drug as aspirin or paracetamol. NSAIDs work by reducing the inflammation caused by an injury – that is, they reduce the swelling, and this reduces the pain because the tissues are not irritated and stretched by the swelling; and this also reduces the damage that can be caused to the cells. This means there is less damage to heal, and when pain is controlled the horse is less stressed, and both these factors speed up healing. If your horse must not move around, this is best achieved through careful management such as bandaging and box rest, rather than immobilizing it through pain.

WHAT YOUR VET MAY DO

Initial examination will involve palpation of the affected limb combined with a series of lameness tests to isolate the area where the damage is most likely to be. Ultrasound scans can then be used to assess the degree of damage and the rate of healing; your vet may choose to scan both legs, as there is often a similar smaller injury in the same position on the opposite leg. The initial ultrasound image can also give a guide as to the likelihood of a return to work, depending on the degree of injury present and the changes that have occurred within the tendon. Your vet will also give you advice on the use of pain relief and supportive bandaging, which are vital for your horse's recovery – but the most important factor in his regime is strict rest. Chronic inflammation or adhesions remaining within the tendon sheath (*tenosinovitis*) once the body of the tendon has healed may be treated by the injection of long-acting steroids.

NEW TREATMENTS

Two recently developed treatments are currently being assessed by the leading equine hospitals. Shockwave therapy involves a low energy soundwave being used to stimulate blood flow to the affected area to help speed healing. Stem cell therapy involves injecting stem cells directly into the damaged area of tendon; the stem cells rapidly form new tendon fibres, and reduce scarring.

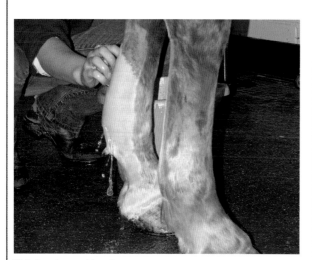

This is a bowed tendon

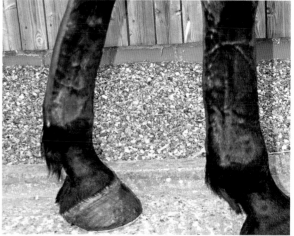

Scarring down the back of the leg is a result of firing to treat a damaged tendon. The leg is clipped and shows signs of current tendon injury

WHAT CAN GO WRONG?

Many tendon injuries heal with rest and time, but the level to which the horse can be exercised and competed may be restricted as the healed tendon will often be weaker and more prone to injury than it was previously.

Complete rupture, particularly of the deep digital flexor tendon, may be irreparable, and in this case your vet may recommend euthanasia.

'Old Wives' Tales'

'MYTH':
Firing a damaged tendon will result in a stronger tissue structure.

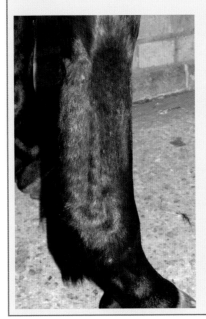

VET'S REPLY:
Tendon firing is an old-fashioned and outdated technique used to treat tendon injuries. The firing process is now illegal in many countries. The theory behind the treatment was that the application of red hot irons to the strained tendon would cause deep burns resulting in scar tissue formation, and this scar tissue was believed to be stronger than the original tendon structure. In reality the prolonged period of rest that was required for the burns to heal also allowed the damaged tendon to heal properly, and scar tissue has now been shown to have only 80 per cent of the strength of healthy tissue one year after an injury.

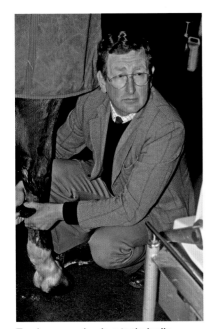

Tendon scanning is a technically difficult investigative technique

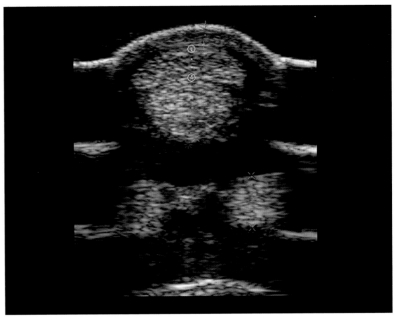

A typical image produced by ultrasound scanning of the flexor tendons

TENDON SHEATH AND BURSA INFECTIONS

FIRST AID FACTS

As with joint capsule infections, tendon sheath and bursa infections are very serious and have the potential to cause permanent damage.

The tendon sheath surrounding the deep digital flexor tendon is very close to the surface, particularly in the region of the pastern, and it is therefore most vulnerable to injury.

Fistulous withers and *poll evil* are infections of the bursa (adapted tendon sheath) which covers the spine at these vulnerable points.

WHAT TO LOOK FOR

- There may be a small injury in the area around the pastern or fetlock.
- Heat and swelling, particularly in areas where tendons are close to the surface, such as the back of the pastern, point of the elbow, poll, withers or hock.
- The horse will be lame, or unwilling to use a limb.

WHAT TO DO

- If you suspect infection in a tendon sheath, call your vet as it will require immediate intensive treatment.
- Cold hosing the affected area can help to ease the pain until your vet can visit.

WHAT YOUR VET MAY DO

This is a very serious condition, like infection in the joint capsule, so your vet may refer your horse to a more specialized clinic for assessment and treatment. Samples will be taken from the affected area to check the nature of the swelling, to confirm if the tendon sheath is involved, and to identify the bacteria causing the infection. This information will give the grounding for formulation of a treatment plan.

Infection of the tendon sheath of the deep digital flexor tendon is very serious and is likely to require referral to a clinic or hospital for intensive treatment. This is likely to include flushing the tendon sheath under general anaesthetic, and injecting strong antibiotics into the tendon sheath. In some cases an indwelling catheter may be placed to allow continued flushing without the need for further anaesthesia.

Infection of the bursa over the withers or the poll is usually treated by flushing with sterile saline and instilling antibiotics. This condition is less serious than a tendon sheath infection because the bursa acts as a cushion and so there is little movement within the bursa, and the formation of scar tissue has less effect.

WHAT CAN GO WRONG?

If scar tissue forms between the tendon and the tendon sheath it limits the range of movement of the affected limb, and will cause both pain and lameness.

If the infection cannot be controlled, the horse may never return to athletic function, and in the worst cases may require euthanasia.

Pain caused by fistulous withers and poll evil may mean the horse is unwilling to be tacked up in the future, as it remembers the pain the tack caused in those areas.

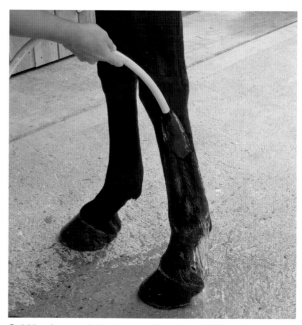

Cold hosing can help to ease the pain until the vet arrives

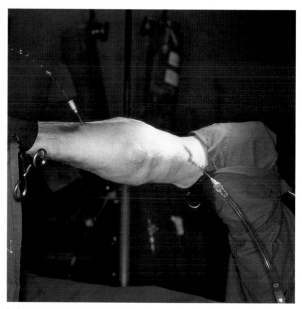

Infections in the tendon sheath require flushing in sterile conditions under general anaesthetic

MUSCLE INJURIES

FIRST AID FACTS

Muscles have a large number of blood vessels so will bruise severely if traumatized; this bruising causes swelling and pain, which will seriously restrict movement.

Wounds deep enough to affect the muscles will bleed profusely because of the number of blood vessels: although this can look quite alarming it can be beneficial as it ensures that plenty of the body's natural healing resources are present at the injury, enabling it to heal more quickly.

80 per cent of muscle wasting happens in the first two weeks of a limb being rested; to help control this, and to help build the muscles back once recovery is complete, physiotherapy under the guidance of a qualified practitioner can provide enormous benefits.

WHAT TO LOOK FOR

- *Deep lacerations* will be obvious, and will be the result of a trauma, for example a fall or running through a fence. There is usually blood everywhere, and the horse will be quite shocked and in pain. It may not wish to put the affected limb to the ground.
- *Bruising* is not always immediately obvious; it usually results from a disagreement with another horse in the field, or from bumping into something hard. A swelling or tender patch, often only noticed when grooming or tacking up, is the initial indicator, although at exercise you may notice that your horse is unbalanced.

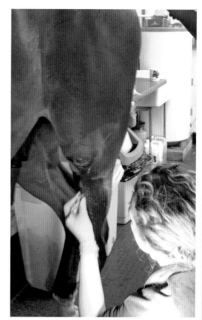

Wound being sutured

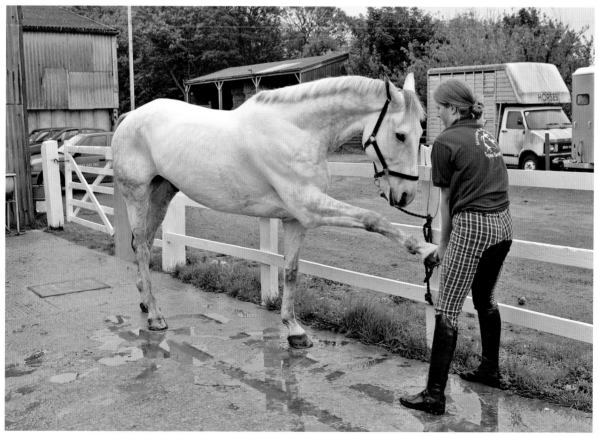

Physiotherapy plays an important role in recovery from muscle injury

WHAT TO DO

- *Deep lacerations* should be flushed quickly with clean, cold water to reduce the pain and to flush any debris from the wound; then apply pressure with clean (ideally sterile) swabs to reduce bleeding.
- You will need to call your vet, as this type of severe wound will require suturing.
- *Bruising* usually resolves in its own time (generally within a week) without any help.
- If your horse is tender, then you can use either a cold compress or cold hosing to reduce the swelling associated with the bruise.
- If the bruising is making your horse lame, then you should call your vet.

WHAT YOUR VET MAY DO

Lacerations: These usually require thorough flushing with sterile saline and checking for foreign bodies within the wound. Once the wound has been cleaned and investigated, then the muscle can be sutured, usually in several layers for extra strength. Antibiotics and pain relief will usually then be prescribed. With serious wounds your vet may recommend a physiotherapist to help with recovery once the superficial injuries have healed.

Bruising: The initial examination will confirm if the swelling is a bruise, or if there is another underlying cause. If there is evidence of infection then antibiotics will be started; if not, pain relief will be given, and advice on massage or physiotherapy to speed up healing.

WHAT CAN GO WRONG?

If wounds heal slowly and cause scarring in the muscle, then movement of that muscle will be reduced and performance may be affected.

Deep wounds in muscles are prone to infection, in part because there is a high risk of debris being left deep in the wound to act as a focus of infection, which may take a prolonged course of antibiotics to resolve.

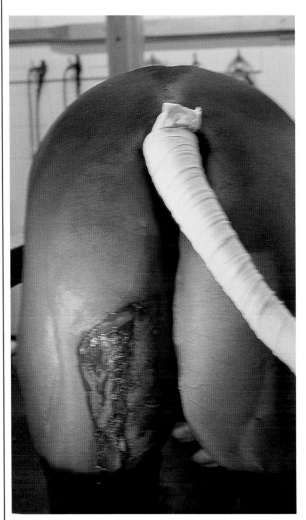 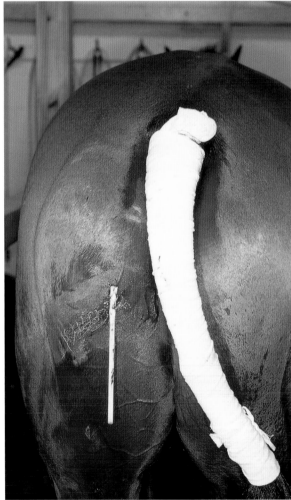

This deep wound into the muscles of the back leg looks very severe: it is closed together with very careful suturing. A drain is being used to prevent the build-up of fluid within the wound, which would slow down healing

A CAST HORSE

FIRST AID FACTS

A horse may become cast through illness, poor stable design, or simply bad luck. What often happens is that the horse lies down normally but then becomes trapped, either getting its legs stuck or not having enough room to stretch its legs to stand properly; this usually happens at night so the horse may struggle all night and become exhausted. A similar effect occurs if a horse falls into a ditch or pond, often worsening its situation by struggling.

In either of these cases ropes and a great deal of care should be used to help the horse out. If you are having problems, or are concerned that the horse has injured itself, the vet should be called immediately, otherwise it is worth calling the vet once the horse is released to check it over and administer pain relief.

WHAT TO LOOK FOR

- The horse is found in the stable lying down, sweated up, very distressed and unable to rise on its own. Also, there are usually signs of a prolonged struggle.
- Usually the horse is stuck in a corner or too close to a wall to be able to extend its legs in order to position itself to rise.

WHAT TO DO

- A cast horse should be approached with caution, as flailing legs from a panic-stricken horse can cause very serious injury to you.
- Wear your hard hat to protect yourself.
- Only approach the horse from behind its back, NEVER between its legs.
- Using ropes or lunge reins around the lower part of the legs closest to the ground, and with the help of at least two other people, pull the horse over on to its other side so that its legs are towards you and it has enough room to get to its feet – and then get out of the way quickly (*see* diagrams, page 92).
- If it is very tired, the horse may not stand immediately, but as long as it can sit in a comfortable, normal-looking position, offer it some hay and water and give it half an hour's peace and quiet.
- Once your horse is standing it should be encouraged to walk around slowly in a soft area to allow circulation to return to the muscles.
- Ideally a cast horse should be checked over by a vet, once it has stood up, to ensure there is no injury, and so it can be prescribed pain relief for its tired muscles.
- The vet should be called if you cannot move the horse.

WHAT YOUR VET MAY DO

If the horse is very stressed or dangerous to handle, then a short-acting sedative may be used to make moving it safer. You may then be able to use different tactics so the horse can move to a position where it can stand up.

Once the horse is moved, the vet will then check it over thoroughly for cuts, scrapes and other injuries, and will then treat any injuries accordingly. Usually cast horses appear quite well when they first stand up, but their bodies become more painful as time passes due to the amount of effort put into trying to stand up – a bit like people overdoing it at the gym! The vet may therefore prescribe painkillers.

WHAT CAN GO WRONG?

There is often an underlying reason why the horse has become cast – for example, rolling because of colic, or because he is stiff and arthritic – which will need to be addressed once he is standing.

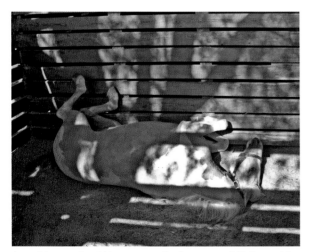

A cast horse should be approached very carefully to avoid injury to yourself

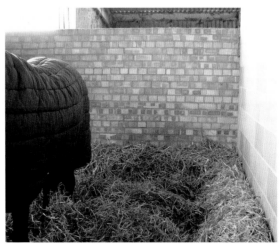

A deep bed with well banked sides will help protect your horse if it becomes cast

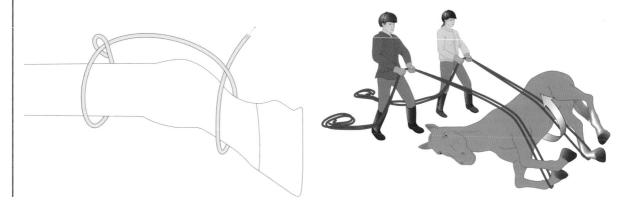

Using ropes or lunge reins around the lower part of the legs closest to the ground, and with the help of at least two other people, pull the horse over on to its other side so that its legs are towads you and it has enough room to get to its feet

If the horse has struggled for a long time while down there may be other soft tissue injuries to the tendons, or cuts and abrasions.

If the horse has been lying in one position for a prolonged period and unable to move, there may be damage to the muscles caused by its weight, because the blood supply to certain areas will have been restricted. This can cause severe pain and significant complications, including sufficient muscle damage that the horse is unable to stand.

CAPPED HOCK / ELBOW

FIRST AID FACTS
A capped hock or elbow is the term used to describe a soft, subcutaneous swelling at the point of the hock or the elbow. It occurs following a direct blow or pressure to the point of the hock or elbow.

WHAT TO LOOK FOR
- A firm, non-painful, immobile swelling on the point of the joint.

WHAT TO DO
- Rest your horse until the acute swelling has decreased.
- Check the swelling regularly for heat and pain.
- If your horse is also lame, consult your vet for advice.

WHAT YOUR VET MAY DO
There is no treatment required other than cosmetic surgery. In acute cases, anti-inflammatories and supportive bandaging may help reduce the degree of swelling. If this is ineffective, or large volumes of fluid are present, then drainage via a sterile needle may be performed; in some cases long-acting steroids may be injected into the tendon sheath to try and prevent further fluid build-up.

X-rays are usually only taken if lameness is also present, as this condition rarely causes lameness; however, the underlying joints are both vulnerable to injury.

WHAT CAN GO WRONG?
Depending on the cause of the swelling there may be an underlying injury, although this is uncommon.

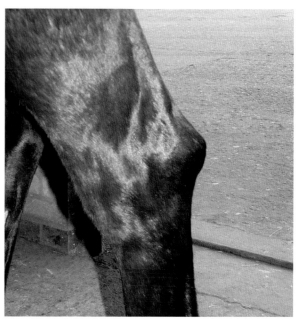

A classic example of a capped hock

WINDGALLS

FIRST AID FACTS
'Windgall' describes a swelling around or just above the fetlock originating in either the joint capsule or the tendon sheath. It is a very common finding on show jumpers because of the extra pressure that is put on the front legs when landing from a jump.

WHAT TO LOOK FOR
- A firm swelling, as described above, which does not cause lameness and often decreases with exercise. The swelling is usually of equal size on both sides of the tendon just above the fetlock joint.

WHAT TO DO
- No action is necessary.

WHAT YOUR VET MAY DO
There is no treatment necessary.

WHAT CAN GO WRONG?
In some cases the appearance of windgalls may affect the sale of your horse, but this is uncommon.

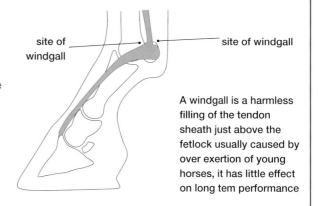

site of windgall

site of windgall

A windgall is a harmless filling of the tendon sheath just above the fetlock usually caused by over exertion of young horses, it has little effect on long tem performance

---

BACK PAIN

FIRST AID FACTS
Pain in the back muscles can cause lameness and poor performance, including an unwillingness to jump. It can also lead to behavioural problems, including bucking and difficulty when tacking up.

WHAT TO LOOK FOR
- Loss of impulsion, or unwillingness to come on to the bit.
- Uneven gait, or unwillingness to move between gaits.
- A sudden unwillingness to have the saddle on, or to be mounted.
- Working unevenly, being unbalanced on one rein.
- Suddenly starting to buck, especially after jumping.

WHAT TO DO
- Run your hands firmly along either side of the spine: pain in the back muscles often shows up as either flinching or muscle tremors when pressure is applied to the affected area.
- Stand behind the horse and check that the muscle shape and size is equal and balanced on both sides of the body and the hindquarters.
- If you think your horse has back pain, consult your vet; depending on the severity of the pain your vet may recommend different types of treatment.

WHAT YOUR VET MAY DO
If your horse is in severe pain, or if there is some lameness apparent, then your vet will recommend a physical examination to try and pinpoint the cause or causes. It is likely that you will be recommended to rest your horse until the condition has been addressed: normally this will be field rest, as gentle movement helps prevent further spasms in the muscles.

Some horses may require pain relief to enable treatment to be undertaken, as the muscles may be too painful to manipulate initially.

There are a number of treatments available depending on the severity of the problem, including physiotherapy, osteopathy, shock-wave therapy, and acupuncture. Your vet will advise which is most suitable for your horse, and will usually be able to recommend a qualified practitioner.

WHAT CAN GO WRONG?
Back pain can, as in humans, be a recurring problem. If this is the case with your horse, you will soon learn the early warning signs, or may be recommended to maintain a regular appointment with a therapist.

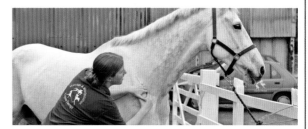

A qualified physiotherapist can help speed the recovery of your horse following muscle injuries

THE FOOT

THE BARE FACTS

The horse's foot and leg are the end result of an evolutionary process designed to maximize their athletic ability. The old adage 'no foot, no horse' is as true today as it has been for hundreds of years, in that most lameness in horses happens as a result of foot problems.

A good farrier is of paramount importance, because poor foot balance can put an excessive strain on tendons, ligaments and joints, ultimately causing pain and injury.

Signs of a healthy foot

- The hoof wall should be smooth, and from the side view, should be at the same angle as the pastern; there should be no cracks, and it should be the same length all round.

- The frog should be smooth and symmetrical in shape, and free from odour.
- The sole of the foot should be smooth and even in colour and texture, and firm to the touch.
- If the foot is too long, this puts too much strain on tendons and joints and can cause pain and lameness; if the foot is too short the sole of the foot may be thin and sensitive, and again it will affect the normal function of the joints and soft tissues.

TOP TIP

Choosing a good farrier is as important as choosing a good vet.

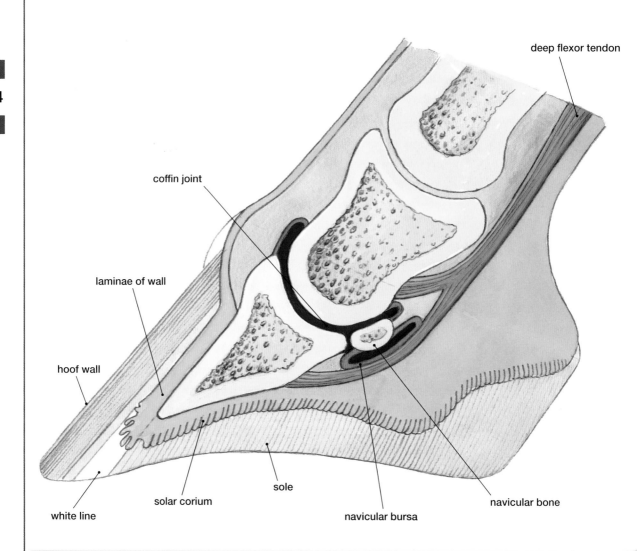

deep flexor tendon

coffin joint

laminae of wall

hoof wall

white line

solar corium

sole

navicular bursa

navicular bone

Conditions affecting the foot

- Acute injury.
- Foot abscess.
- Puncture wound to the sole of the foot.
- Laminitis.
- Thrush.
- Mud fever.
- Shoeing accidents.
- Hoof wall injuries.

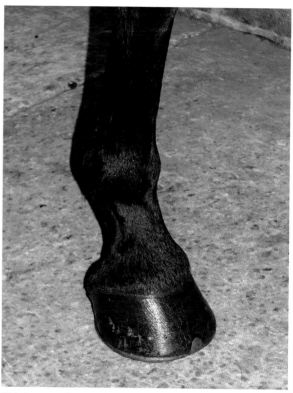

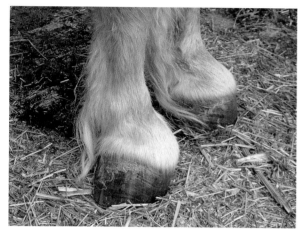

These abnormal feet are produced by a combination of poor conformation and lack of appropriate farriery when this horse was a foal

This is a good example of a normal healthy foot; note that the hoof wall and pastern are at the same angle and the hoof is symmetrical

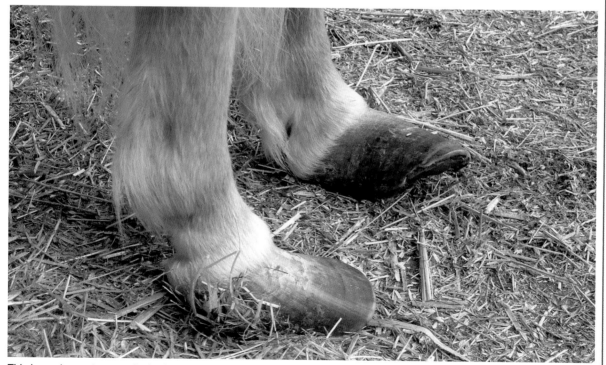

This horse has not seen a farrier for over a year; as a result the hooves have grown so long the flexor tendons have become stretched, so correction will need to be carried out very carefully

ACUTE INJURY

FIRST AID FACTS

Acute injury to the foot is quite common, and can easily happen in the field or out on a hack.

Wire injuries around the pastern and fetlock (or rope injuries in tethered horses) can look to be purely superficial; however, the joint capsule and digital flexor tendon sheath are quite close to the skin, so any wound in this area – particularly if the horse is suddenly very lame – should be examined extremely closely. If you are in any doubt, call your vet.

WHAT TO LOOK FOR

- Check for any sign of injury to the foot, pastern or fetlock area.
- If the horse is suddenly lame with no apparent external injury, then suspect pus in the foot or possible damage to the joint capsule or tendon sheath.

WHAT TO DO

- Injuries around the foot, pastern and fetlock should be cleaned immediately and inspected to see how deep the wound is.
- Superficial wounds can be treated with a topical antiseptic if they are shallow and no important structures are involved.
- If you are worried, or if your horse is more lame than you would expect, call your vet.

WHAT YOUR VET MAY DO

Injuries around the pastern and fetlock will be carefully investigated to ensure that neither the joint capsule nor the tendon sheath has been damaged.

If the injuries are purely superficial, then sutures may be placed, depending on how extensive the injury is, and antibiotics and/or pain relief prescribed. However, if there is a suspicion that the joint capsule or tendon sheath has been affected, then immediate hospitalization and intensive treatment will be required. This usually involves high doses of antibiotics and intensive flushing of the affected structure.

WHAT CAN GO WRONG?

Wounds in this area, even if small or shallow, can be difficult to keep clean and free from infection; careful management is needed, combined with bandaging if this is appropriate.

Both the joint capsule and the tendon sheath are very close to the surface of the skin, particularly around the back of the pastern. Injury to the joint capsule or tendon sheath can be very serious, particularly if infection develops, and without aggressive intervention can lead to irreparable damage.

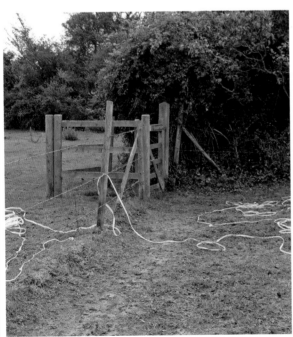

Electric fencing left loose on the ground can easily become caught around the foot or pastern, potentially causing deep lacerations to this vulnerable area

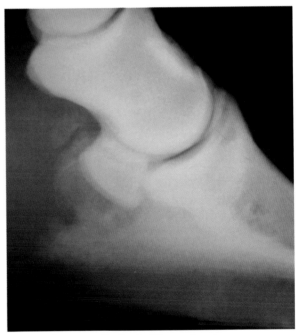

Arthritic change on the front of the pastern bone

FOOT ABSCESS

FIRST AID FACTS

A foot abscess can be caused by a puncture wound, bad shoeing, a bruising to the foot, or chronic seedy toe. The intense pain is caused by the build-up of pus within a restricted area, putting pressure on sensitive tissues.

WHAT TO LOOK FOR

- Often the first sign of a foot abscess is finding your horse suddenly extremely lame and unwilling to put the affected foot to the ground despite no obvious injuries.
- The digital pulse, felt either on the fetlock or pastern, is a very good indicator of inflammation in the foot. The more inflammation there is in the foot, the stronger the pulse feels. This is particularly useful for monitoring a foot abscess.
- Bruising can sometimes be visible on the sole of the foot; it is made more obvious by cleaning the foot thoroughly first.
- Smell is also a good indicator of foot health: if there is a draining abscess there is a characteristic smell; thrush also has a very individual smell.
- An abscess will often only show as a small black dot on the sole of the foot, sometimes with a soft area of sole around it.

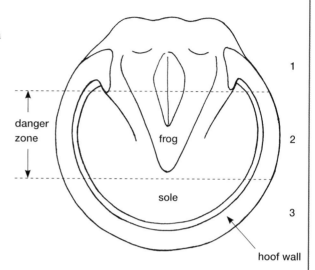

The danger zone, marked above, is the area of the sole where penetration by a foreign object is most likely to cause serious damage, such as hitting the navicular bursa or the pedal bone

CHANGES IN THE CORONET BAND

The coronet band should be smooth and level with the top of the hoof wall. A change in position of the pedal bone within the hoof, such as is seen with severe laminitis, can cause a dip all the way around the top of the hoof (right). An abscess in the foot can sometimes work its way up inside the hoof and burst through at the coronet band, and this will also show initially as a softening in the coronet band – but normally only in one area rather than all the way around (bottom). An abscess that bursts out of the coronet band can be very difficult to clear up because the drainage is against gravity, so it may need poulticing or antibiotics, and it definitely needs advice (though calling for advice does not necessarily mean a visit).

Basically, if you notice either of these changes, call your vet for advice.

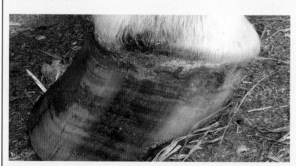

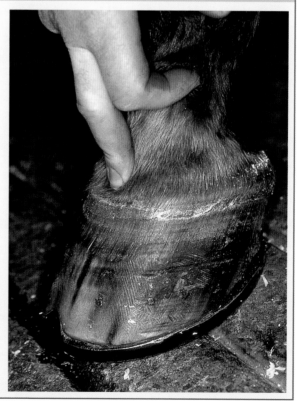

WHAT TO DO

- If your horse is suddenly very lame and unwilling to put a foot to the ground you should call your vet.
- If you think your horse's foot smells unusual, clean it thoroughly to find the source of the smell.
- If you suspect an abscess, call your vet or your farrier for advice.

TOP TIP

Some horses have very hard soles, and this can make it extremely difficult to explore the foot; in this case a wet poultice kept on the foot for as long as possible before the vet or farrier arrives may help to soften the sole and facilitate examination.

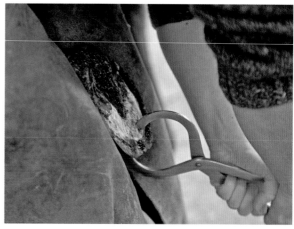
Hoof testers are used to locate the painful point in the foot

WHAT YOUR VET MAY DO

A foot abscess usually requires further exploration of the foot to find its root; either your vet or your farrier can do this. In many cases the foot is so painful that it cannot be investigated without pain relief, sedation and sometimes even a local nerve block.

Once the location of the abscess has been confirmed and the area cleaned as much as possible, a poultice will be applied. This is usually soaked in hot water, and great care must be taken when applying it to the foot to ensure the heel is not scalded; the poultice is then bandaged in place and secured using either tape or a protective boot.

Some vets give antibiotics, while others prefer not to: this decision is made depending on where the abscess is, and how badly affected the foot is. Antibiotics are more likely to be prescribed for an abscess which has burst out of the coronet band, as this is a deeper seated infection which may not resolve with poulticing and natural drainage alone.

WHAT CAN GO WRONG?

An unchecked abscess can track up from the sole of the foot and burst out through the coronet band; this is intensely painful. The severe pain can make the horse unwilling to bear weight on the affected foot, which can lead to damage to the soft tissues on the opposite leg caused by excessive weight-bearing. A support bandage should therefore be applied to the opposite leg and adequate pain relief given to allow the horse to bear some weight on the affected limb.

98

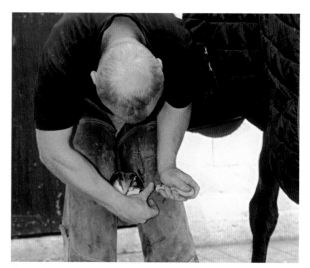
Once the pain has been localized, careful paring with a knife will locate the exact point of the abscess

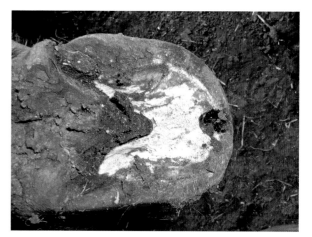
The tip of the toe is a common site for a foot abscess to develop; however, once the pus starts draining the horse recovers quickly

PUNCTURE WOUNDS TO THE SOLE OF THE FOOT

FIRST AID FACTS

Puncture wounds to the sole of the foot can also affect vital structures, depending on the position of the puncture wound on the sole of the foot. There are generally few repercussions in the outside 2–3cm (¾–1in) around the diameter of the foot; however, any injury close to, or involving the frog or heels should be treated seriously, as deep penetration of a puncture wound can involve the pedal bone, navicular bone or the deep digital flexor tendon sheath.

WHAT TO LOOK FOR

- Any type of foreign body that may have entered the sole of the foot, for example a nail or toe clip from a dislodged shoe, particularly in the event of sudden onset acute lameness.

WHAT TO DO

- If you find a nail or some other sharp object in the sole of your horse's foot, clean the area immediately around the object and then, using your fingers or some pliers, pull it out slowly and mark the foot clearly to show where it was: then call your vet.
- Unlike a foreign body in another part of the body, it may be necessary to remove an object stuck in the sole of the foot if the horse is attempting to bear weight on that leg, as this will drive the foreign body deeper into the foot and make it more likely to cause serious injury.
- Do not throw the foreign body away as it is important for the vet to see what it is, and how big it is.
- Put a protective pad over the foot to prevent any dirt getting into the wound while you are waiting.
- If the shoe is half pulled off remove it carefully, if possible; if not, remove any nails pulled out of the foot, replace the shoe in its normal position and secure with self-adhesive bandage or tape until professional help can be obtained.

TOP TIP

Removing a shoe is difficult; next time your farrier is shoeing your horse, watch carefully and ask for a demonstration on how to safely remove a hanging shoe.

WHAT YOUR VET MAY DO

Treatment depends on the nature and size of the foreign body, and how deeply it has penetrated the sole of the foot. For a small or shallow wound the vet will give your horse antibiotics to fight infection, use antiseptics to clean the wound, and offer advice as to the best way to poultice and treat the wound in order to promote healing as efficiently as possible.

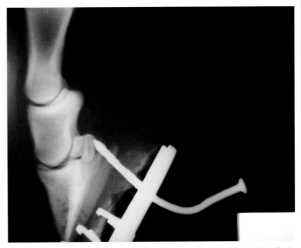

A serious penetration of the foot with a foreign body (nail): it is touching the navicular bone, and will be embedded in the deep digital flexor tendon

If the vet feels the wound needs further investigation – for example the foreign body is still lodged in the foot, there is a complicated laceration, or the puncture wound is in the sensitive central portion of the foot – then the horse may be sedated or local anaesthetic used to examine the injury. General anaesthesia will only be suggested in serious cases.

Any puncture wound in the central portion of the foot has the potential to affect vital structures, and in these cases x-rays will be taken to assess the depth and position of the injury. If the pedal bone, navicular bone or navicular bursa have been affected, then aggressive treatment will be required to control infection.

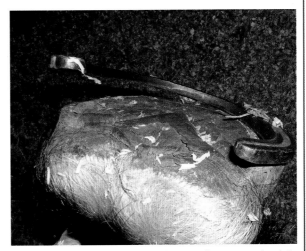

A loose shoe like this either needs removing or securing into a normal position until a farrier or vet can remove it properly

Puncture wounds are the ideal environment for tetanus infection to develop, so if there is any doubt regarding the continuity of the horse's tetanus vaccination programme, a tetanus anti-toxin injection may be given so as to ensure that the vaccination status is up to date.

WHAT CAN GO WRONG?

Despite initial antibiotic treatment, pus in the foot can still develop. Moreover, damage to any of the vital structures found in the foot (pedal bone, navicular bone, navicular bursa or the root of the deep digital flexor tendon) can have serious consequences and a poor prognosis for recovery to soundness.

LAMINITIS

FIRST AID FACTS

Laminitis is an extremely painful condition which can lead to euthanasia if it is poorly controlled. It is characterized by inflammation of the laminae which help secure the pedal bone in position within the hoof capsule; when this inflammation is severe the laminae become detached and the pedal bone can drop out of position, resulting in chronic lameness.

The inflammation is very painful because the laminae are trying to swell and cannot because of the hard hoof wall; this causes a sensation very similar to the throbbing pain of a bruise under the fingernail.

The most commonly recognized cause of laminitis is overgrazing on lush pastures, particularly in native ponies. Fructan, a type of sugar, has been implicated in laminitis cases related to overgrazing, as levels of this sugar are abnormally raised in lush grass. In these cases an imbalance in the bacteria of the hindgut caused by the excessive levels of carbohydrate (sugars) means that too much of this sugar is absorbed.

It is not only lush grazing that can cause a bout of laminitis (although this is the most common cause): problems associated with foaling, severe infection (**septicaemia**), Cushing's disease, and pressure from lameness on the opposite foot can also cause laminitis.

WHAT TO LOOK FOR

- Digital pulses, felt either on the fetlock or pastern, are a very good indicator of how much inflammation is present in the foot. The more inflammation in the foot, the stronger the pulses feel; this is particularly useful for monitoring the development and recovery of laminitis.
- The coronet band should be smooth and level with the top of the hoof wall; abnormal movement of the pedal bone can cause a dip here (*see* box, page 97). If you notice this, call your vet immediately.
- Laminitis usually develops in at least two feet together; normally the front feet are affected first, although this is not a firm rule.

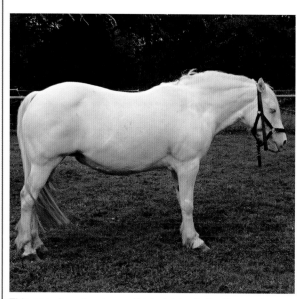

This pony is a classic candidate for laminitis; the cresty neck and fat pads around the body are indicators of equine metabolic syndrome

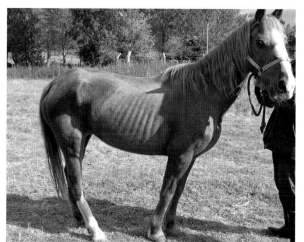

This pony has been on a restricted diet as a result of a bout of laminitis, but this was not done under the supervision of a vet, and the pony is seriously underweight. Very careful dietary management will now be required in order for it to regain condition while avoiding laminitis or diarrhoea

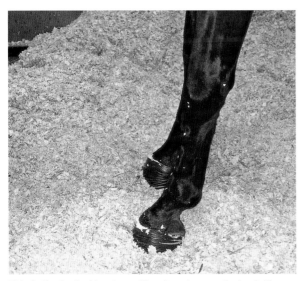

This is the typical backward leaning stance of a laminitic horse

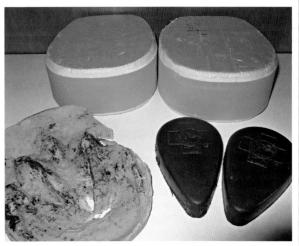

There are various different supports available for the frog and sole of the laminitic horse, the one used will depend on the severity of the condition and the preference of the vet

- Initially your horse may be sound over soft ground such as grass, but not willing to walk over gravel or concrete; furthermore, as the laminitis progresses, even moving on soft ground will become painful.
- Further progression will cause the horse to lean back on to its heels in an attempt to take the pressure off its sore toes.

101

TOP TIP

Horizontal rings on the hoof wall are evidence of previous bouts of laminitis where the normal growth of the hoof wall has been disrupted.

IMPORTANT POINTS OF DIETARY MANAGEMENT FOR LAMINITIS

1. Low levels of dietary carbohydrates: this means that any foods containing sugars (such as sugarbeet) or wheat, oats or barley should be avoided.
2. High levels of fibre: hay, haylage, chaff and so on.
3. Restricted grazing: this can be achieved either by restricting the grazing to a very small area, using a grazing muzzle, or by turning out the horse in a manège with a haynet.
4. Mineral and vitamin supplementation: this is important in ponies that have their diet closely restricted.

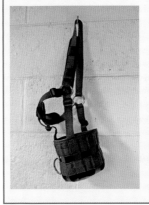

A grazing muzzle restricts the total grazing of the horse wearing it, and only allows the tips of the grass to be grazed: these contain lower levels of the sugars that are thought to be involved in the development of a laminitic episode

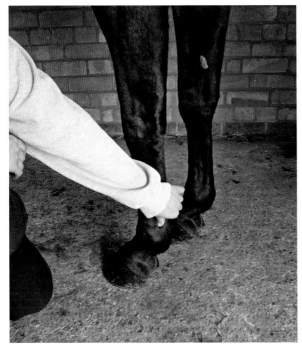

Monitoring the strength of the digital pulse can help indicate inflammation in the foot

WHAT TO DO

- Bring your horse in immediately, preferably into a stable with a thick deep bed of shavings all the way up to the door, and call the vet if this is the first time this horse has been affected.
- The deep shavings will pad the soles of the feet and spread the horse's weight slightly. If you are unable to do this, then padding the feet with cotton wool slippers (*see* Bandaging, page 26) will give your horse some measure of relief.
- Long-term management of a chronic laminitic horse varies between individuals and is best planned in conjunction with both your vet and your farrier following initial treatment.

WHAT YOUR VET MAY DO

When laminitis is suspected, pain relief is given quickly; it is usually given in conjunction with a **vasodilator**, which helps to reduce the pressure in the foot. Depending on the severity of the laminitis, foot supports can be fitted either by the vet or the farrier to support the pedal bone and reduce the risk of it rotating.

X-rays may be taken to assess the position of the pedal bone within the hoof, usually if the lameness is severe or if there have been repeated bouts of laminitis. Remedial farriery also makes use of the x-ray images to plan corrections to help the recovery process.

Dietary management is very important, particularly as this disease is most commonly seen in fat native ponies; your vet will advise you as to the best way to manage your horse. This primarily will involve restricting carbohydrates, and restricting grazing, though inevitably advice will be tailored to the individual.

WHAT CAN GO WRONG?

Poor ongoing management following a bout of laminitis can lead to recurrent bouts of the disease, and this could result in a gradual rotation of the pedal bone.

In the worst case scenario the rotation of the pedal bone can lead to it breaking through the sole of the foot. This condition is untreatable and results in euthanasia of the horse or pony.

CUSHING SYNDROME AND LAMINITIS

The extremely long haircoat in the photo is typical of Cushing syndrome (see page 151), and is usually accompanied by a strong tendency to develop laminitis.

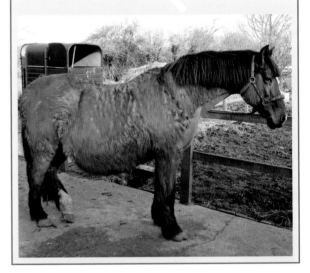

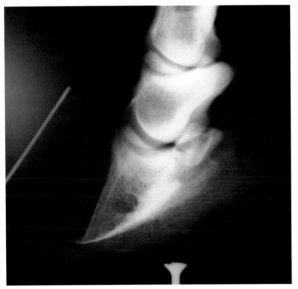

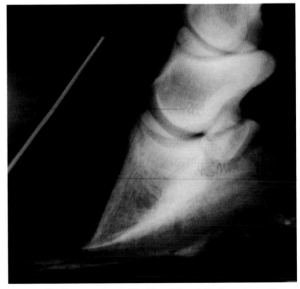

Both these feet show rotation and dropping of the pedal bone as a result of severe laminitis. The thin white line above the pedal bone is a lead marker on the hoof wall, and should be parallel with the angle of the pedal bone

THRUSH

FIRST AID FACTS

Thrush is generally a mild, self-limiting yeast infection of the skin, which is located mainly on the sole of the foot. It is most commonly seen when the weather is unrelentingly wet and the animal is left out in the mud and the sole of the foot has been unable to dry out properly.

WHAT TO LOOK FOR

- Smell is always a good indicator of foot health: thrush has a very individual, unpleasant smell that will come from the infected area.
- Thrush usually occurs around the heels and frog: there may be some swelling or oozing in this area, and the surrounding tissue is usually soft and soggy.

WHAT TO DO

- Pick the foot out, then clean and wash the foot with an antibacterial and/or antiseptic wash at least twice a day.
- Dry the foot and try to prevent the horse from getting its feet wet for long periods of time.
- Continue to treat the foot until the smell has gone.
- Call your vet or your farrier for advice.

WHAT YOUR VET MAY DO

This condition does not normally require veterinary involvement; however, in extreme cases pain relief or stronger topical treatments may be prescribed.

WHAT CAN GO WRONG?

If the initial infection is not controlled, then secondary bacterial infection can also develop.

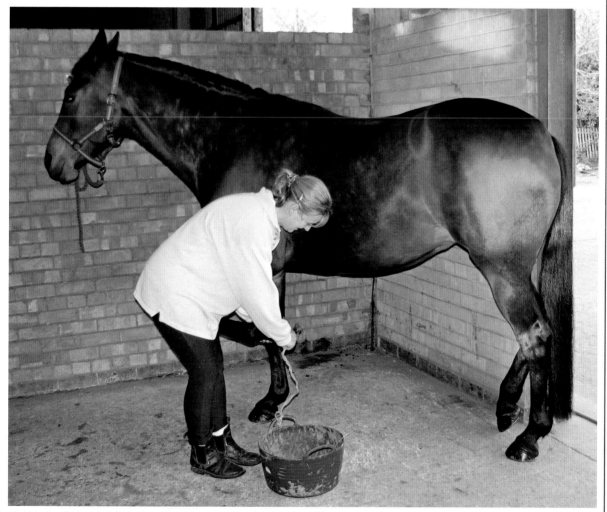

Picking the feet out daily is important to maintain a healthy foot. Thrush tends to develop in feet which remain packed with stable manure for prolonged periods since it maintains a moist environment and encourages the growth of yeasts

SHOEING PROBLEMS

FIRST AID FACTS

Ill-fitting shoes, or shoes left on the foot for too long, can lead to pressure on the hoof horn causing swelling and bruising: this is known as a corn. Corns can cause low grade, intermittent lameness as well as sudden lameness. A nail prick is when a nail is driven too close to the laminae and puts pressure on the sensitive white line, causing acute onset of lameness.

Over-trimming of the hoof wall at shoeing may cause immediate lameness. Continual over-trimming or under-trimming will upset the balance of the foot, with knock-on effects on the surrounding soft tissues, potentially causing a continuing lameness.

An overgrown toe is more prone to develop white line disease. This is where the layer between the outer and inner hoof wall is weakened by stress, potentially allowing foreign material, such as gravel, to penetrate the hoof wall and set up infection. This may cause sudden onset lameness.

WHAT TO LOOK FOR

- If your horse resents a nail being driven in, it is possible that a sensitive part of the foot has been irritated; sometimes there will be bleeding following the removal of the nail.
- Your horse should be comfortable immediately following shoeing; if it is sore, the shoe may have been nailed on too tightly (too close to the sensitive laminae) or the hoof wall has been trimmed back too severely.

WHAT TO DO

- If your horse is lame following shoeing, ask the farrier to remove the shoe from the affected foot.
- If you suspect a nail bind or prick, soak the foot in an antiseptic solution and then keep it clean and dry for the next 24 hours. If the penetration is deep, then call your vet for advice.
- If removing the shoe does not relieve the problem, call your vet.

A GOOD SHOEING JOB

- The angle of the hoof wall should be in line with the angle of the pastern.
- The hoof walls should be symmetrical and even in length when the foot is picked up and then viewed from the heels.
- All nail heads should be sunk into the shoe to prevent early wear, and the cleats (the sharp ends of the nails) should be knocked down and smooth with the surface of the hoof wall.

TOP TIP

You should only use a farrier who is fully qualified and registered with the Honorable Company of Farriers, or a supervised apprentice.

WHAT YOUR VET MAY DO

Once the lameness is located in the foot, hoof testers are used to localize the point of pain within the foot (see photo page 98); this area can then be investigated with a hoof knife to locate the source of pressure and release it. Once the source of the pain has been addressed, then either a poultice or protective dressing or padding can be applied to protect the sole of the foot (see page 24).

In cases of known deep penetration of the sole, antibiotics may be prescribed in combination with pain relief, or if the central portion of the foot has been affected, then X-rays may be taken to check for the involvement of vital foot structures.

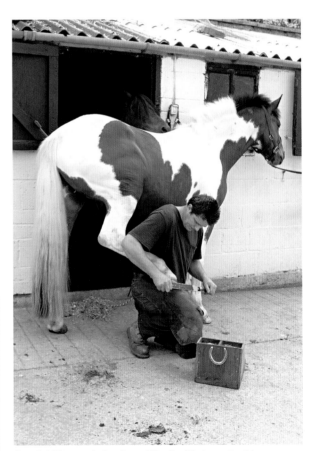

Careful filing and shaping of the foot is important to maintain good hoof horn quality

WHAT CAN GO WRONG?

In the long term, poor foot balance can lead to chronic lameness resulting from inappropriate strain being placed on the soft tissues of the leg.

Ill-fitting shoes can also lead to the development of corns, which can cause sudden onset lameness, as well as long-term, intermittent lameness.

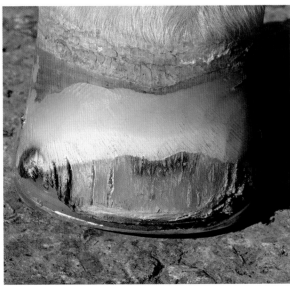

Changing the balance of the foot by shortening the toe can improve the horse's recovery from a bout of severe laminitis

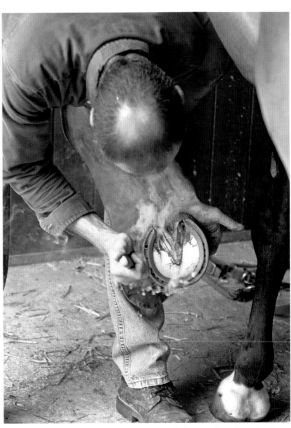

Hot shoeing allows a more precise fitting of the shoe to the horse's foot

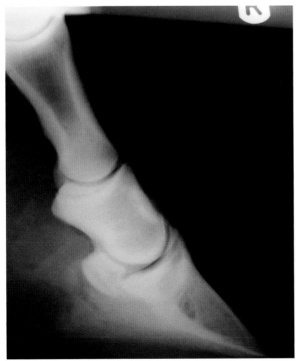

A normal angle of the pedal bone, pastern and canon bone in relation to each other

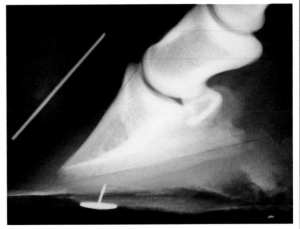

An abnormal position of the pedal bone: the drawing pin in the sole of the foot should be level with the tip of the pedal bone, and the pastern bone should be at the same angle as the pedal bone

HOOF WALL INJURIES

FIRST AID FACTS

The quality of the horn produced varies between individuals, but is also affected by the quality of nutrition being fed. Supplementation, primarily with biotin, can help to improve the quality of the new hoof. The rate of growth in an average horse is approximately 1cm (½in) each month – at this rate an entirely new hoof wall is grown in around nine months.

WHAT TO LOOK FOR

- Cracks, either horizontal or vertical, that are deepening or lengthening.
- Irregularities in the smooth surface of the hoof wall – this might be a tumour involving the horn of the hoof known as a keratoma, but this is rare.

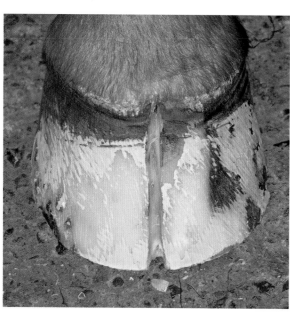
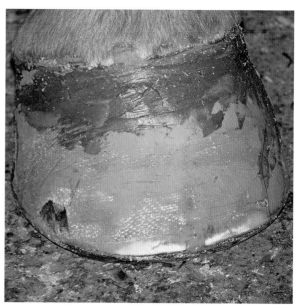

This hoof has a vertical crack running from the coronet band to the bottom of the hoof wall. To prevent this causing problems, such as the hoof wall collapsing or infection entering the foot via the crack, the crack has been drilled out and then the hoof wall supported and protected with a treatment of specialized resins

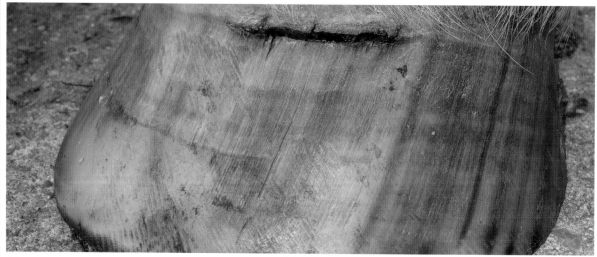

A horizontal crack in the hoof wall is less serious than a vertical crack, only becoming a problem as it nears the ground when it may cause a large portion of hoof wall to break away

WHAT TO DO

- Any injury that penetrates the hoof capsule requires immediate attention.
- Put a protective dressing over the injury to protect the hoof from further contamination.

WHAT YOUR VET MAY DO

Initial assessment of the injury will probably involve x-rays of the foot to check for deeper damage. Injuries and deep cracks to the hoof capsule can be strengthened and supported with either metal plates or special resins until the affected area of the hoof has grown out. Long-term treatment will involve close liaison between your vet and your farrier to achieve the best results. With careful support the damaged area of the hoof will grow out, leaving a normal foot.

WHAT CAN GO WRONG?

Severe damage to the hoof capsule can result in permanent deformity and chronic lameness.

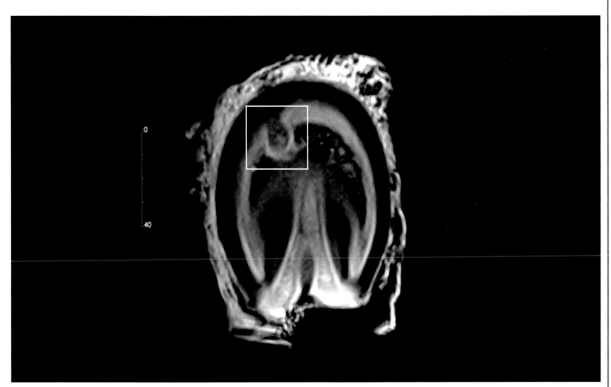

An MRI image of a keratoma (a hoof wall tumour) which puts pressure on the inside of the foot

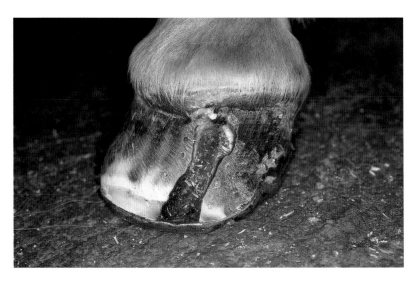

The keratoma is removed by aggresively drilling away the affected hoof wall to ensure no abnormal tissue remains. It will now be covered with a resin to strengthen the hoof capsule and prevent contamination until the drilled area grows out

THE SKIN

THE BARE FACTS

The skin is the largest single organ in the body. Fair-skinned horses are as prone to sunburn as fair-skinned people, and although a horse's skin is quite tough, it is as prone to injury and allergic reaction as our more delicate human skin.

Thoroughbred horses have much thinner, more sensitive skin than native and cob types, but both have problems that are specific to their skin type. In the same way, some horses are much more sensitive to fly and insect bites.

Signs of healthy skin
- Healthy skin is smooth and elastic.
- Coat hair should be smooth and shiny, and even in texture and length.

Conditions affecting the skin
- Traumatic injury (open wounds).
- Urticaria (fly bites and allergic skin reactions).
- Mud fever.
- Parasitic attack (lice, sweet itch, ringworm).
- Sunburn and photo-hypersensitivity.
- Cellulitis (swollen limbs).
- Haematoma (bruising).
- Sarcoids and melanomas (skin cancer).
- Eye problems.

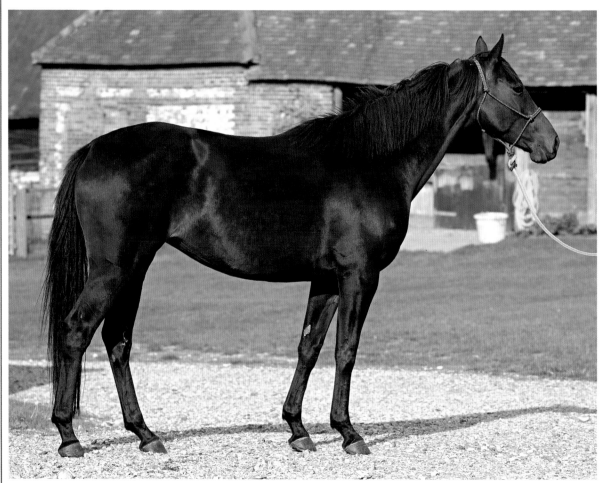

Thoroughbred horses have much thinner, more sensitive skin than native cob types

TRAUMATIC INJURIES

These injuries include grazes, cuts and puncture wounds.

FIRST AID FACTS

Horses can injure themselves in an empty field, so they should be checked for injuries at least once a day.

This whole topic is covered in more detail in Part 1 'Dealing with Wounds', *see* page 14.

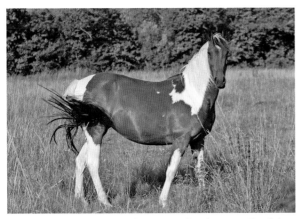

Biting insects cause many horses to develop an urticarial reaction, one of the most common skin complaints

URTICARIA

FIRST AID FACTS

An allergic reaction is an over-reaction by the immune system to foreign material – such as insect saliva from fly bites, or contact with certain plants.

Urticaria is the nettle rash-style inflammation that usually results from fly bites or contact allergies, and it is often intensely itchy; in rare cases the horse's immune system will react so violently to a bite or skin irritant that the horse will begin to have trouble breathing and will rapidly develop shock-type symptoms (known as *anaphylaxis*) – in this instance call the vet immediately.

WHAT TO LOOK FOR

- A reaction to fly bites is characterized by small, localized lumps, often quite tender to touch and which may ooze clear or bloody fluid. They may occur singly, or in groups.
- An allergic skin reaction may cause small lumps over the skin where the horse's skin has come into contact with the irritant.
- Urticaria is similar in appearance to the rash caused on human skin by nettles – usually a large number of swellings of varying size, or intensely itchy bumps on the skin.

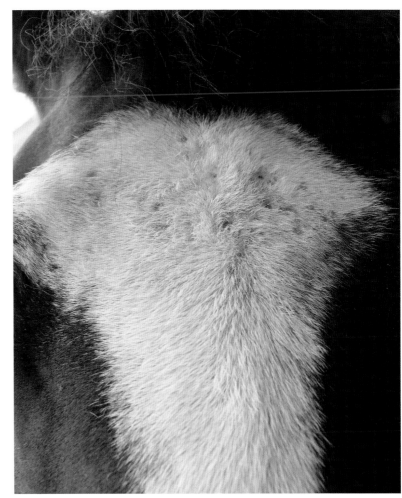

The hair loss on this horse's face is the result of an allergic reaction to fly bites

WHAT TO DO

- Cold hosing can give some relief from itching if the horse is distressed.
- Soothing creams and ointments can be applied if the bite is itchy or oozing; the type of product used is generally a matter of personal preference. Any product that contains a soothing compound and/or antiseptic is fine (such as insect bite creams that are available over the counter).
- Take care to use padding if the affected area comes into contact with tack or harness.
- Call the vet if the bite or skin reaction develops into an urticarial reaction and/or your horse is breathing more quickly than normal, is finding it difficult to breathe, or seems very distressed, as it may be experiencing a severe allergic reaction.
- If your horse is very itchy and is scratching to the point of injuring the skin further, then veterinary treatment may be required to relieve the itching and prevent further injury.

WHAT YOUR VET MAY DO

In severe allergic cases where your horse is having problems breathing or is injuring itself while trying to scratch, your vet may administer some drugs to relieve the symptoms. These may be anti-histamines or steroids, depending on the severity of the problems and your horse's clinical history.

Long-term medical treatment may be required to prevent recurrent episodes. Specialized skin tests can be used to identify the exact cause of the allergic reaction, so than an individual vaccine for your horse can be developed to desensitize it to its allergens.

Changes in how you manage your horse may be recommended to reduce the risk of further episodes. This can include changing the time of day or place of turnout, and the use of specialized rugs, as well as changes to bedding and feedstuffs.

WHAT CAN GO WRONG?

Self-trauma (scratching) can damage the skin, and infection can develop. In very rare cases anaphylaxis can be followed by death if this allergic condition is not recognized and treated quickly.

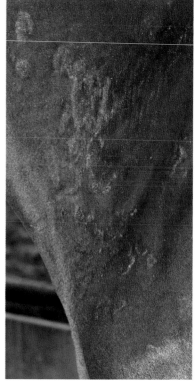

Self-trauma can complicate the treatment of skin conditions

110

TOP TIP

Bites which are under the tack can be rubbed and develop secondary infections, so a thick layer of extra padding should be used if you have to place tack over a bite.

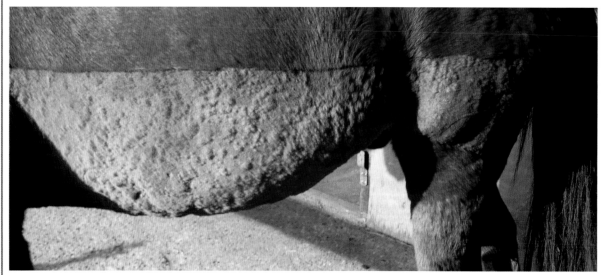

Severe urticarial reaction

MUD FEVER

FIRST AID FACTS

Mud fever is generally a mild, self-limiting bacterial or yeast infection of the skin, located mainly on the pastern. It is most commonly seen in heavy horses with feathering, because the longer hair can keep these areas quite moist and warm – and these are ideal conditions for microbes to grow in. Mud fever can be seen at any time of the year, but is more prevalent when the weather has been very wet.

WHAT TO LOOK FOR

- Look for sore skin patches, and cracks, bleeding or scabs in the pastern area.
- In severe cases the affected areas may spread up the leg causing more serious problems, such as cellulitis.

WHAT TO DO

Mild cases of mud fever may be successfully treated in the following way:

- Cut away any hair that is covering the sore area.
- Clean and wash the area with an antibacterial and/or antiseptic wash.
- Pick off any scabs; this will uncover any yeast/bacteria that are growing there.

- Dry the area thoroughly and cover with an antibacterial and/or antiseptic cream.
- Continue to treat the area until all the scabs have gone and the skin has healed.

WHAT YOUR VET MAY DO

There is rarely any need for veterinary involvement other than for cases that are extensive or are not responding to basic treatment.

In these stubborn cases antibiotics can be given either in feed or as a topical cream; some horses may also need pain relief, particularly if the leg swells in reaction to the infection. In extremely stubborn cases samples may be taken and sent to a laboratory for culture and sensitivity tests.

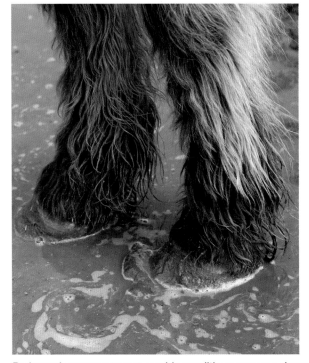

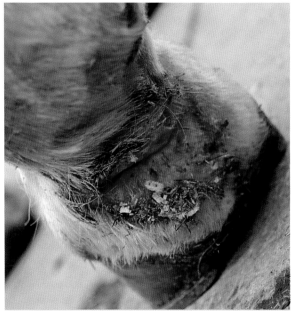

Prolonged exposure to wet, muddy conditions causes a dermatitis of the pastern and fetlock region commonly known as mud fever

PARASITIC ATTACK

FIRST AID FACTS
- Lice are more commonly found than people will admit.
- Sweet itch is an allergic reaction to the bites of the *Culicoides* midge.
- Ringworm is a fungal skin infection that is highly contagious for both horses and humans.
- Harvest mites (*Trombicula autumnalis*) are a seasonal problem, usually affecting the face and legs.
- Mange is uncommon.

WHAT TO LOOK FOR
Lice
- Usually the first signs are extensive areas of dandruff; as the infection spreads, small white lice can be seen on closer examination of the hair.

Sweet itch
- Classic signs of sweet itch are areas of the mane and tail rubbed raw.
- In chronic severe cases there is thickening of the mane and tail area even in the winter.

Ringworm
- Ringworm patches are not necessarily round! They can appear anywhere on the body, but are most commonly seen in areas that have contact with tack and harness.
- Initially you may notice tufts of hair that are clumped together, and a slight thickening or swelling of the skin underneath. The hair then falls out, leaving the underlying skin sore and raw.
- In chronic cases the affected skin is grey and flaky, with broken hairs surrounding the patch.

Harvest mites and mange
- The most common symptom is itchiness, usually shown by leg stamping, head shaking and repeatedly rubbing the affected areas.
- Small scabs will develop, and these are often accompanied by hair loss.

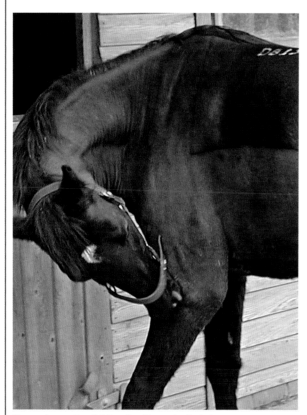

If your horse is nibbling itself, particularly in response to grooming, it means that it is very itchy – often because of a skin mite or louse infestation

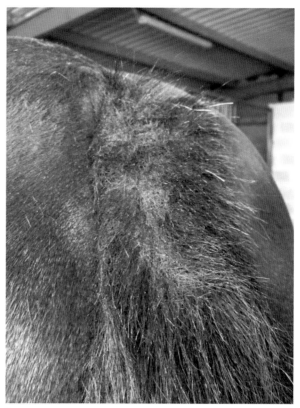

This rubbed tail is typical of the early stages of sweet itch

WHAT TO DO

Lice
- There are a number of lice powders on the market, the important active ingredient being *permethrin*. Any product containing this compound is adequate to treat this condition effectively.
- Call the vet if the lice do not respond to treatment, as there may be an underlying disease that is making your horse vulnerable to parasites.

Sweet itch
- Where possible, prevent the horse coming into contact with biting insects, either by using rugs or changing grazing patterns.
- Care should be taken and extra padding used for sore areas that come in contact with tack or harness.
- Soothing creams and ointments can be applied if the area is itchy or oozing. The type of product used is generally subject to personal preference. Any product that contains a soothing compound and/or antiseptic is fine.
- Call the vet if you believe the reaction is becoming severe, and the horse is distressed.

Ringworm
- If you suspect ringworm, call your vet as this condition can be passed on to other horses, other animals and people, so it needs prompt diagnosis and treatment.
- Remember to take extra caution with your personal hygiene, because you could catch it.

Harvest mites and mange
- If you suspect mites or mange, contact your vet to confirm the diagnosis and instigate the most appropriate treatment.

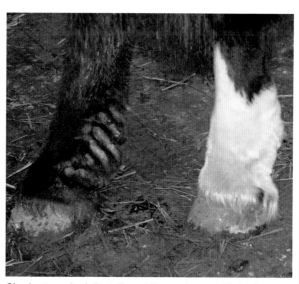

Chorioptes mite infestation of the pastern and fetlock

WHAT YOUR VET MAY DO
So as to confirm the diagnosis your vet will probably take samples of hair and scrapings from the skin to examine under the microscope. This should show up fungi, bacteria and ectoparasites (lice or mites); these samples may need to be sent away to a specialist laboratory if confirmation of the diagnosis is needed.

Blood samples may be taken if there is a suggestion of underlying disease that is contributing to the condition. Once a firm diagnosis has been made, then a suitable treatment programme can be instigated.

WHAT CAN GO WRONG?
In some horses susceptibility to ectoparasites is related to a weakened immune system, and may be an indicator of underlying disease. Where recurrent infestations occur, or the condition is resistant to treatment, then further medical investigations for systemic disease are indicated.

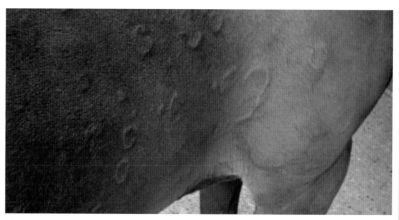

These lesions can be a bacterial or fungal skin infection

SUNBURN AND PHOTO-HYPERSENSITIVITY

FIRST AID FACTS

Pink-skinned areas, such as flesh marks and the back of the fetlock where there is little protective hair, are vulnerable to sunburn. Sun-block cream should be used here to protect the skin from damage during the summer.

Another reaction to light can occur with certain types of poisoning and chronic liver disease; this is known as photo-hypersensitivity. The areas most vulnerable to this condition are the same as for sunburn, but it will also extend into any white-haired areas. The skin blisters and peels, and the surrounding area will swell up in a manner similar to cellulitis. If this happens, call your vet.

WHAT TO LOOK FOR

Sunburn

- Sunburn looks much the same on a horse as it does on people.

Photo-hypersensitivity

- Photo-hypersensitivity causes the skin to blister and peel, with very little exposure to the sun.
- Swelling and blistering occur in white-haired areas where the skin is not directly exposed.

WHAT TO DO

Sunburn

- With sunburn, cover the area with a sun lotion that is designed for children or animals, both to soothe and protect the horse from further sun damage. Continue this until the weather cools down, or the risk of sunburn has decreased – much as you would with your own skin.

Photo-hypersensitivity

- If you suspect photo-hypersensitivity, call the vet.

WHAT YOUR VET MAY DO

Sunburn

In severe cases the vet will administer painkillers to reduce the discomfort, and will advise you on how best to treat the burns with appropriate topical applications.

Photo-hypersensitivity

The vet will advise you to keep the horse out of any direct sunlight until the underlying condition is diagnosed. Usually blood samples are taken to check for evidence of liver or other organ problems, and treatment is then started accordingly.

WHAT CAN GO WRONG?

Photo-hypersensitivity is nearly always the result of severe underlying disease, usually affecting the liver. This condition may be difficult to treat.

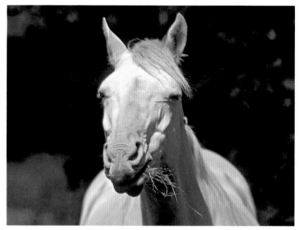

A pink face like this is very prone to sunburn, so preventative measures should be taken

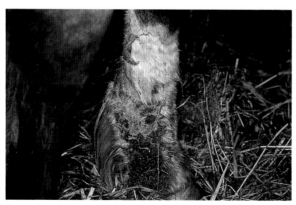

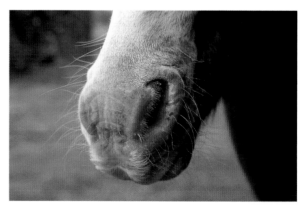

Acute liver failure makes the non-pigmented areas of skin vulnerable to burning and blistering, a condition that can be easily confused with sunburn. The two photographs above are of horses that had the appearance of sunburn despite relatively low levels of exposure to the sun, on further investigation both had serious liver disease

CELLULITIS AND LYMPHANGITIS (SWOLLEN LIMBS)

FIRST AID FACTS

Cellulitis is the name given to describe inflammation of the connective tissue found just below the skin, most usually seen in the lower limbs of the horse surrounding a wound or point of injury. The inflammation and swelling is generally due to a powerful reaction of the immune system to a bacterial infection.

The lymph drainage system runs in parallel to the circulatory system: when it becomes inflamed it is referred to as lymphangitis, and is most commonly caused by an injury on the lower limb introducing infection into the lymph system. Sporadic lymphangitis can develop in horses that are left standing in the stable for prolonged periods of time; this is when there is swelling that comes up overnight despite there being no injury. The hind limb is more commonly affected than the forelimb because of a difference in the pattern of the lymph vessels between the front and back legs.

Cellulitis can be difficult to differentiate from lymphangitis; cellulitis normally develops immediately around the site of injury, with the fluid then following gravity and filling up from the bottom of the leg. Lymphangitis is a failure of the lymph drainage, and so the leg will fill from the bottom up.

WHAT TO LOOK FOR

- The leg appears thickened and loses all definition.
- The limb is hot and painful to the touch.
- There may be fever and the horse may be off colour.
- In severe cases there may be some oozing from the surface of the skin (cellulitis) or ulceration (lymphangitis).
- The horse is often lame on the affected leg.

WHAT TO DO

- In mild cases, where only a single lower limb is affected and the horse is not lame, cold hosing is often effective. This should be repeated at least twice a day on the leg(s) until the swelling goes.
- Cellulitis is usually an over-reaction by the local immune system to infection, so check the affected leg thoroughly for any injuries, including mud fever.
- Where there is mild thickening of the limb and no severe lameness your horse will benefit from being turned out, as movement of the limb encourages both the circulation of the blood but also improves the movement of the lymph.
- If the horse is lame or the skin appears taut, call the vet, as your horse may need medication.

WHAT YOUR VET MAY DO

If there is a suspicion of infection, then antibiotics are often prescribed and anti-inflammatories given to reduce the swelling. If there is an obvious and/or infected wound, then a swab may be taken to allow for bacterial culture to enable more accurate use of antibiotics.

WHAT CAN GO WRONG?

Severe cellulitis can lead to serum oozing through the skin, which in turn scalds the superficial tissue, thus exacerbating the condition. This chemical burn must be treated in the same manner as a thermal burn, and likewise can be difficult to treat.

Severe lymphangitis caused by bacterial infections can lead to ulcers developing on the affected limbs, which then become susceptible to infection in their own right.

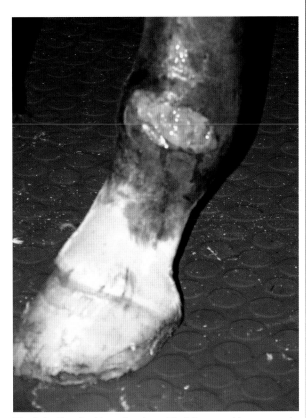

The infection that has developed in this wound has caused the limb to swell above the wound: this is the early stages of cellulitis

HAEMATOMA (BRUISING)

FIRST AID FACTS
Haematoma is the medical term for a bruise, which is characterized by a firm painful swelling. The swelling is caused by broken blood vessels, leading to bleeding under the skin.

WHAT TO LOOK FOR
- A firm swelling at the site of a severe blow – for example, a stifle injury when a horse has caught its hind leg on a jump, or following a kick injury if the skin has not been broken.

WHAT TO DO
- In mild cases, cold hosing is often effective. This should be repeated at least twice a day over the affected area until the swelling resolves.
- Avoid exercise until the lump has reduced in size.

- If the size of the lump increases you should contact your vet, because there may be an infection developing in the haematoma.

WHAT YOUR VET MAY DO
Large haematomas can be very painful, so once the vet is happy that the swelling is simply a haematoma, pain relief may be prescribed. If there is a wound overlying the haematoma, or other risk of infection, then antibiotics may also be prescribed.

WHAT CAN GO WRONG?
Most haematomas heal without complications, though in some cases scar tissue may form which may leave uneven tissue. The pain of the haematoma may mask an underlying injury which will only become apparent once the haematoma has resolved.

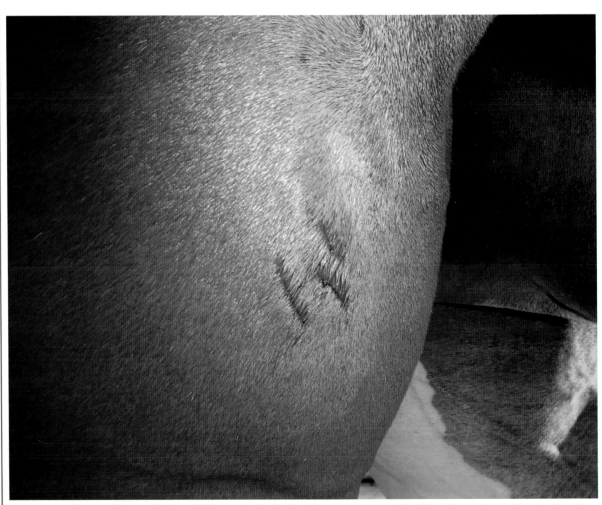

This horse fell into a ditch, and although it has sustained only minor scrapes over the stifle, a haematoma has developed

SARCOIDS AND MELANOMAS (SKIN CANCER)

FIRST AID FACTS

Sarcoids and melanomas are forms of skin cancer that are specific to horses. Both types are benign in that they do not spread and form secondary tumours elsewhere in the body. However, they can grow rapidly, and multiple tumours can arise spontaneously.

Sarcoids are believed to be caused by a viral infection in a manner similar to warts or cold sores. Bovine papillomavirus type 1 or 2 is thought to be involved, although exactly how, is still unclear.

Melanomas are only seen on grey horses and are thought to be the result of melanin (skin pigment) abnormalities. Most grey horses will begin to develop melanomas by approximately 15 years of age.

WHAT TO LOOK FOR

Sarcoids

- Sarcoids are most commonly found on the head, especially around the eyes, on the legs and on the abdomen – particularly between the back legs.
- Sarcoids are normally slow-growing and should not be itchy.
- There are five main types of sarcoid:
  - **Fibroblastic**: ulcerated, and similar in appearance to proud flesh.
  - **Nodular**: smooth lumps with normal skin.
  - **Occult**: crusty, scaly, lichen-like lesions.
  - **Verrucous**: warty in appearance.
  - **Mixed**: a combination of fibroblastic and verrucous types of sarcoids.

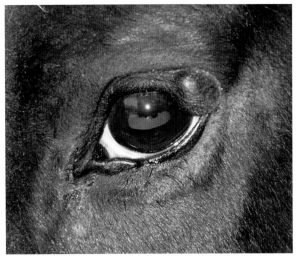

This is a typical site for sarcoids to develop on the face; in this position removal can be difficult

VIRAL WARTS

In horses under three years old, warts often appear on the muzzle, ears, eyelids, lower limbs and genitalia. These normally disappear within two to three months, and should not be mistaken for sarcoids.

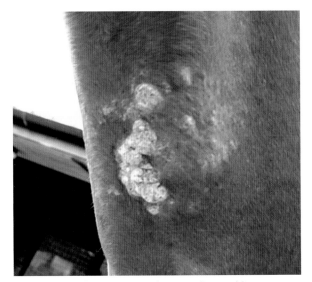

This is a typical appearance of an occult sarcoid

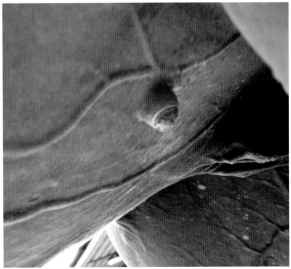

The groin is a classic position for the development of sarcoids; this is a nodular sarcoid

Melanomas

- Melanomas are usually smooth-shaped lumps that generally appear around the tail, under the dock and around the anus; however, they can develop anywhere on the body.
- They are very rarely malignant other than when they arise in non-grey horses.
- Clinically, a melanoma will cause few problems unless the position is underlying the tack, where it may rub.
- In some cases, as the horse gets older, numerous tumours may develop around the anus, and these can prevent the normal function of defecation, which will lead to secondary infections.

WHAT TO DO

Sarcoids

- If you suspect your horse has a sarcoid, call your vet for further advice.

Melanomas

- These are not serious initially; show them to your vet on a routine vaccination visit, unless the melanoma is interfering with either the tack or with normal function (such as defecation).

WHAT YOUR VET MAY DO

Sarcoids

There are many treatments available to try and remove sarcoids and to prevent their recurrence. Successful treatment normally depends on the type of sarcoid and its position – and these factors influence the type of treatment chosen. Treatments available include surgical treatment, normally backed up by cryosurgery or cauterization, and also the use of topical toxic creams, or possibly the injection of the BCG vaccination directly into the sarcoid.

Melanomas

Where treatment is necessary, surgical removal is the normal course of action. Samples can be taken from lymph nodes to assess if there is the potential for further development of tumours in the short term. Melanomas often develop in groups and are slow-growing, so surgical removal is rarely called for.

Recent developments have included the use of an anti-histamine to control the rate of growth, and the manufacture of a desensitization vaccine from a melanoma that has already been removed. Both of these treatments have varying degrees of success.

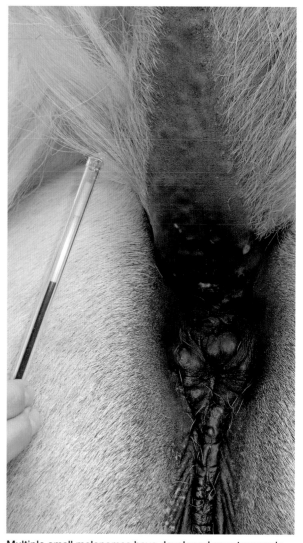

Multiple small melanomas have developed spontaneously on the dock and around the anus and vulva of this mare. This is very common in middle-aged grey horses

EYE PROBLEMS

FIRST AID FACTS

Infections in either the tissue surrounding the eye (conjunctivitis) or the surface of the eye can be extremely painful; if the horse starts rubbing its eye to relieve the discomfort, then it can worsen the situation, so call your vet for advice as soon as you see any abnormality in the shape, colour or general appearance of the eye.

Equine recurrent uveitis, or moon blindness, is a condition where the iris (the coloured part of the eye) repeatedly becomes inflamed and can scar, affecting the way the pupil constricts and reducing the visual field. Inflammation of the iris appears as a darkening or change in colour of this pigmented part of the eye.

WHAT TO LOOK FOR

- Any abnormality in the shape, colour or general appearance of the eye.
- Blinking very rapidly or refusing to open the eye.
- Tears spilling out of the eye and running down the face.
- Conjunctivitis causes the tissue surrounding the eye to become very red and swollen, and causes the eye to run.
- When there is an injury to the cornea the surface of the eye becomes cloudy, and may appear white or blue, and there may be a break in the glossy surface of the eye.
- If there is anything on the surface of the eye which does not move when the horse blinks, then call the vet as this may be a foreign body in the cornea.

TOP TIP

Eye injuries can be very serious: if you think your horse has injured its eye, call your vet immediately.

WHAT TO DO

- If there is a slight reddening of the tissues surrounding the eye and a small amount of discharge, bathe the eye carefully with cooled, boiled water for two days. The eye should improve during this time.
- Call your vet immediately if
  - the surface of the eye seems cloudy and/or white;
  - there is any direct injury (i.e. a laceration) to the surface of the eye or the eyelid
  - there is anything stuck on, or in, the surface of the eye or in the eyelids
  - there is severe inflammation of the conjunctiva
  - your horse is unwilling to open its eye.
- Bring your horse into a darkened stable until the vet is able to examine the eye.
- You may need to protect the eye from further damage: if you have access to a pair of blinkers, these can stop rub or knock injuries. If not, then try and distract your horse by grooming him or by giving him a small concentrate feed.

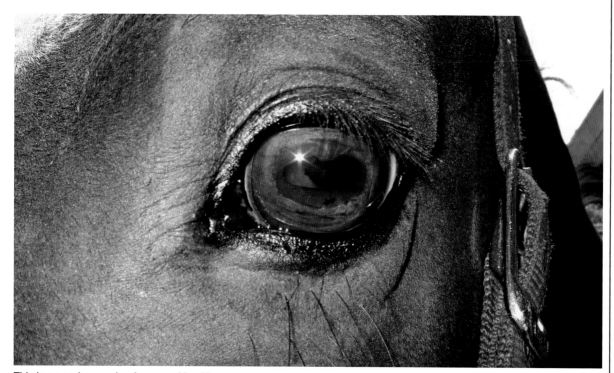

This is a good example of a normal healthy eye

WHAT YOUR VET MAY DO

Where there is severe pain, local anaesthetic eyedrops may be needed to facilitate a fuller examination of the injured eye without distressing the horse further. Fluorescine dye can be used to highlight damage to the surface of the cornea, showing up as a bright green area where there is damage.

Simple infections of the eye can be treated with topical antibiotics, but very badly affected eyes may be treated with a combination of both topical and systemic medication. Horse-sized contact lenses may be used as a bandage to help protect the surface of the eye while it is healing. Severe injuries where the surface of the eye is badly damaged may require surgical correction.

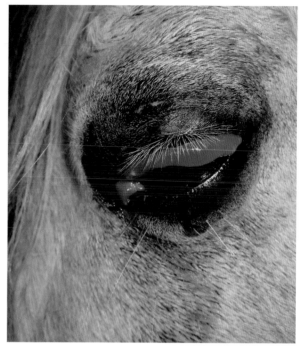

Conjunctivitis is a very painful condition – even mild inflammation can make your horse avoid light and become head shy

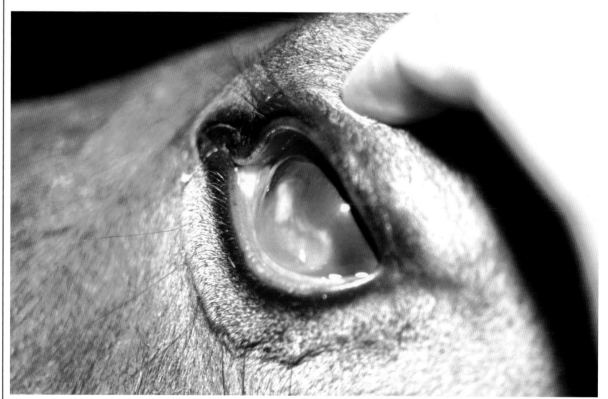

A melting ulcer, such as seen on this pony's eye, can have serious consequences, including rupture of the eyeball or permanent scarring which affects the field of vision. It is very important to seek veterinary attention for any abnormalities on the surface of the eye

WHAT CAN GO WRONG?

Penetrating injuries, such as a puncture wound from a thorn, can cause changes within the eye leading to the development of cataracts and loss of vision in that eye. Severe lacerations to the cornea can lead to the loss of vision in the affected eye, and in worse case scenarios, the eye itself.

Unrecognized moon blindness will lead to scarring of the iris, which stops it adjusting the pupil size in different light conditions; this in turn leads to over-exposure of the retina to light, and consequential damage to the eyesight.

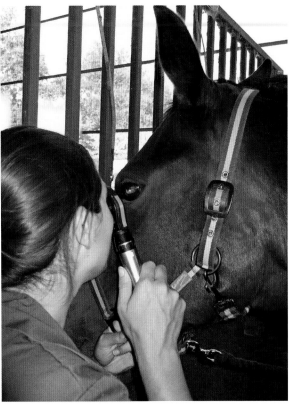

A full ophthalmic examination will include the use of an ophthalmoscope to examine the lens and retina

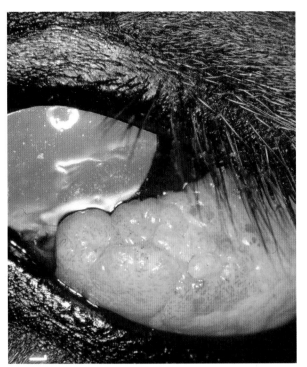

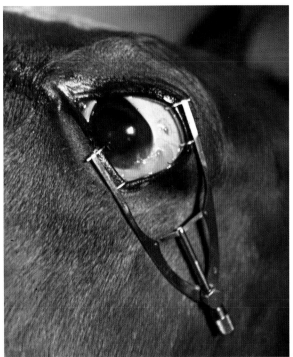

The large growth in the eyelid of this horse is unusual and aggressive. Its removal required a full anaesthetic and radiotherapy, but ultimately was successful

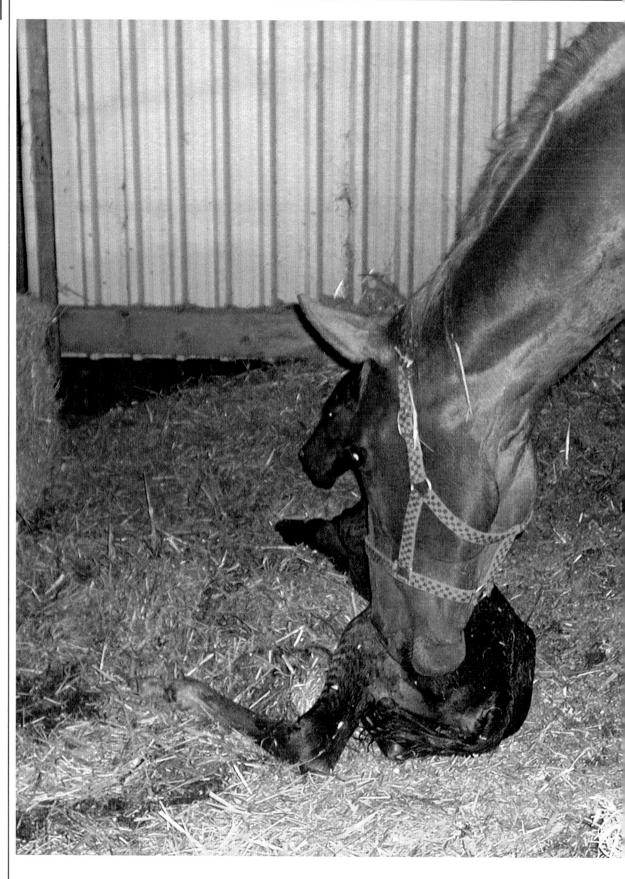

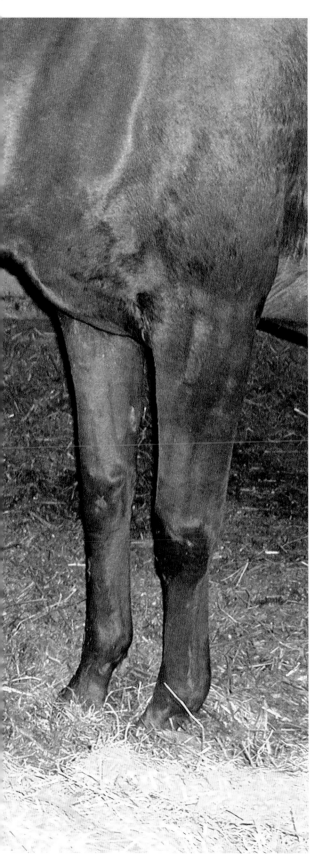

SECTION 3
HOW TO APPROACH EMERGENCY SITUATIONS

This section covers the emergency situations that horse owners dread, explaining how to gain control over events, and helping you to stay calm when it matters most. Each situation is broken down into the areas you need to be aware of, highlighting potential dangers to both you and your horse, and explaining how to avoid these pitfalls and how to decide what course of action to take.

ROAD TRAFFIC ACCIDENT

FIRST AID FACTS
The first priority is to prevent the situation becoming any worse for both the humans and the horses involved in the incident. Any injured people will have to be attended to and taken care of first.

WHAT TO DO
- Make the accident site as safe as possible; enlist bystanders to slow down or stop oncoming traffic where possible.
- Secure any horses, either by tying them to something safe or shutting them in a nearby field or garden.
- Loose horses should be caught up if possible as they have the potential to cause further accidents; however, you must assess if there is a more immediate need to help an injured person.
- Check injured people following first aid principles ('Airways, Breathing, Circulation'), check for consciousness and any obvious sources of pain. Under no circumstances remove the riding helmet: leave this to trained first aiders. If it is possible and safe to do so, move the injured person to the side of the road. If in any doubt call an ambulance immediately.
- Check injured animals following the same first aid principles: injuries can range from bruising to catastrophic, but even with no obvious external injuries horses should be checked over by a veterinary surgeon – even if all that is needed is some pain relief.
- If there is a serious injury and you need to call the vet, try where possible to give the following information as accurately as possible:
  - location;
  - the number of animals involved;
  - if the emergency services are involved;
  - a description of the injury or the condition of the affected animal;
  - If you think euthanasia may be necessary;
- Depending on the nature of the injury, the next priority is to prevent it becoming any worse – for example, apply pressure to a bleeding wound to minimize blood loss.

WHAT YOUR VET MAY DO
Your vet may ask you to organize transport for the affected horse if your description suggests that treatment or admission to a veterinary hospital is necessary, although the horse should not be moved unless it has been assessed as fit to travel by the vet.

When the vet arrives, a thorough assessment of the nature of the injuries will be made, and treatment started according to the clinical findings. Some treatments may be carried out *in situ* – for example, pain relief or suturing small wounds – while others may be better treated either at the stables or the clinic.

TOP TIP
It is an offence to transport an animal in a weak, debilitated state or if it is injured, unless it is under the direction and supervision of a veterinary surgeon.

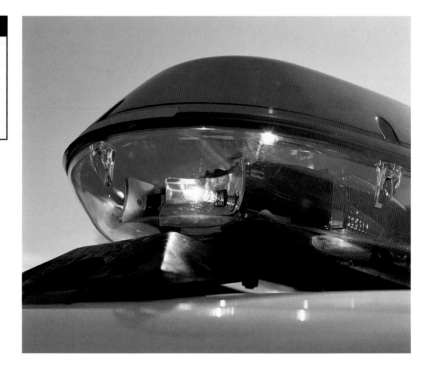

FIRE

FIRST AID FACTS

Human safety is always of paramount importance, so never take risks with your own life for the sake of your horse, or anyone else's.

Note that severe damage can be done to the lungs as a result of smoke inhalation, even when there are no external signs of injury or burns. When the lungs are irritated by smoke inhalation, excessive fluid is produced, which forms a barrier between the alveolar surface and the air, making it difficult for oxygen to be absorbed. Breathing therefore becomes deeper and more rapid to allow sufficient oxygen to be absorbed.

WHAT TO LOOK FOR

- Signs of fire; smoke, either white or black; or flames, most likely in the region of stored bedding, feed or rugs.
- Signs of thermal injury: burns are most likely to be at the extremities, the hair will be singed, and there will be bubbling of the superficial layer of the skin (blisters).
- Damage to the airways and the lungs shows as increased rate and depth of breathing, usually with associated increased noise (wheezes), which becomes gradually worse.

WHAT TO DO

- Call the fire brigade: it may sound obvious, but in your panic your reflex reaction may be to dive straight in; however, you will need professional help.
- Look after your own safety next: alert someone close by to the situation so that they can come and help.
- You should never go into the building if there is no one else around, or if the fire has taken a strong hold.

FIRE SAFETY PRECAUTIONS

- Make sure the yard is a no-smoking area; sand buckets can be used at the entrance to make sure any cigarettes are properly extinguished.
- Each yard should have a clearly displayed fire protocol and evacuation procedure.
- Make sure the yard has the correct number and type of fire extinguishers, and have them serviced regularly.
- Make sure that electrical wiring is checked regularly – at least annually; horse feed attracts rodents and these chew wires, which can start fires.
- If you have a burning muck heap, make sure that it is situated well away from the stables, and downwind of the prevailing wind.
- If you are unsure about the arrangements for your yard, contact your local fire safety officer for advice.

- If you have to go into a smoky stable, use a damp towel to cover your mouth and nose to protect against smoke inhalation.
- You will probably need to cover the eyes and ears of your horse as you lead it out, as it is likely to be panicked by the fire and refuse to move; if it is smoky you should also try and cover its nostrils with a damp towel to protect it from smoke inhalation.
- Once the horses are away from the fire, make sure they are out of the smoke plume and check them thoroughly for injuries.
- The most likely injuries are burns, irritation to the eyes and airways, as well as cuts and scrapes.
- A cold hose or a sponge with plenty of cold water will help to soothe most injuries: use it to flush any cuts or scrapes, or sore eyes.
- If there are burns to the skin, flush it with copious quantities of cold water until the heat in the skin has subsided, then cover with something waterproof – such as clingfilm – until the vet arrives.
- If everyone is out and safe you can attempt to deal with the fire: aim water at the base of the fire, or damp down as much of the unaffected flammable material as possible, but do not put yourself in harm's way.

WHEN TO CALL THE VET

Call your vet as soon as possible: it is likely that your horse will need treatment quickly. You can always cancel the call if you get the horses out very quickly and as long as they are showing no ill effects at all – but it is still better to get them checked over.

Remember that injuries relating to exposure to heat and smoke can take a little time to develop fully, so monitor your horse closely for a couple of hours after exposure, particularly in relation to breathing, as lung damage is very common following exposure to smoke.

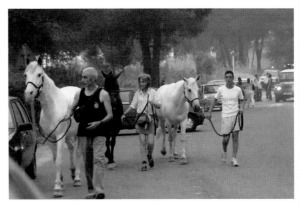

Enlist as much help as possible to calmly lead the horses as far from the fire as practical

CAST HORSE

FIRST AID FACTS

Always be aware that you are at greater risk of injury than your horse if you are not very careful about how you attempt to deal with it while it is cast. Wear a hard hat if possible, to protect your head from wayward kicks.

Your horse is likely to have multiple small cuts and grazes, and will probably be very stiff and sore as a result of becoming cast.

WHAT TO LOOK FOR

- A cast horse is usually stuck on its side or back with its les bent up close to a wall or fence; there may be signs of a struggle, and the horse is usually sweated up and very stressed.
- Check for any obvious reasons why the horse has become stuck, for example colic.

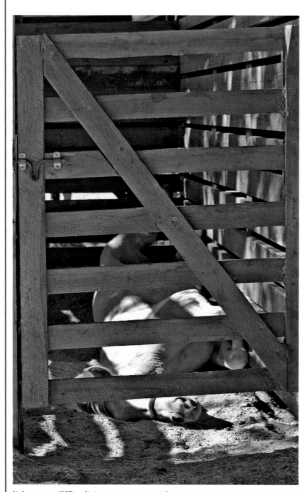

It is very difficult to move a cast horse or even pony on your own. You should get at least two other people to help, and wear your hard hats for protection

WHAT TO DO

- Get some help; it is very difficult to move a horse on your own.
- Collect a couple of lunge reins or very long lead reins.
- If possible find hard hats for you and your helpers.
- Carefully approach the horse from its back; never get in between its legs while it is down.
- Attach the lunge reins to the fetlock and canon bone (see diagram) of at least the front and back legs closest to the ground; you can put ropes on all the legs if you have enough.
- Once you are happy that the ropes are secure, stand as far away as possible and gently pull on them, smoothly and gradually. You are aiming to slowly roll the horse on to its back, and then gradually bring the legs all the way over towards you so that the horse is lying on the opposite side to the way you found it with its legs away from the wall or fence.
- The horse should now have room to draw its legs underneath its body and stand up.
- Once the horse is up, you should check it over thoroughly for any injuries.

WHEN TO CALL THE VET

- If you are not confident to move the horse, or cannot find any help.
- If your horse is unable to stand once it is moved into a position where it should be possible for it to do so.
- If you are concerned that there is a serious underlying illness which has caused the horse to become cast.
- If you find injuries which you are concerned need professional attention.

WHAT THE VET MAY DO

What the vet will do depends very much on the situation they are presented with; however, they have more experience of these situations than you have, so will be able to judge very quickly if more extreme solutions will be required, such as lifting equipment.

If there is an underlying condition that is preventing your horse from rising, this can be addressed.

If your horse has been stuck in one position for a prolonged period the vet may advise you to walk it around, or may suggest some stretches to help the muscles recover more quickly.

HORSE STUCK IN A DITCH OR CATTLE GRID

FIRST AID FACTS

Unless you are very lucky and find your horse shortly after it has become trapped, it is likely to be exhausted and very stressed by the time you do find it. In this situation human safety is paramount, so be very careful as you approach your horse, as it may panic and injure you in its struggle.

Traumatic incidents such as a thunderstorm, or some other terrifying moment, can cause horses to bolt and they risk running into this type of hazard and becoming trapped in these circumstances.

If you think you will need heavy lifting or cutting equipment, begin arranging this as soon as possible. However, be prepared for the worst: horses can readily break a leg in this situation, so a calm approach is vital in order to prevent further injury once you have discovered a horse in such a situation.

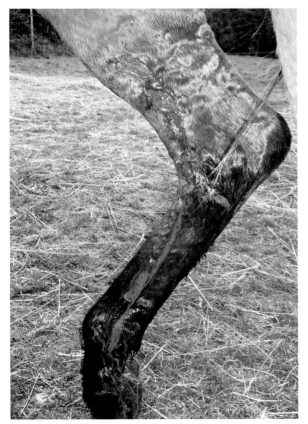

This horse was trapped in a ditch and injured itself while trying to escape, which is why most of the injuries are on the inside of the leg

WHAT TO LOOK FOR

- If your horse is trapped in a cattle grid, check the trapped limbs carefully for any evidence that the bones have been damaged, or that any important structures have been injured.
- If your horse is stuck in a ditch, check to see if any of the limbs are stuck down into the mud, and if the angle that the trapped legs are at is normal.
- Check for any other injuries.
- Monitor the heart rate, breathing rate and the colour of the gums to check for shock and pain.

WHAT TO DO

- Calming the horse down is the most important requirement in this situation; if it is firmly stuck, then panicked attempts to free itself can result in further injury, particularly in a cattle grid. You can offer some water and a haynet, if these are available, to help it calm down and recover its energies.
- If the horse is reacting to equipment arriving to release it, you can put cotton wool in its ears to dull sounds, and in some cases tuck a towel or a sweatshirt over its eyes. If you cover the eyes you must stay in contact with the horse to reassure it.
- You will need to get help, as it is impossible to extract the horse on your own; you are likely to need soft ropes or lunge reins, spades and sacks or blankets if it is in a ditch, and cutting equipment or similar to dismantle the cattle grid.
- Many fire brigades will not attend an emergency involving animals unless a vet is also in attendance, so have your vet's phone number to hand.

WHEN TO CALL THE VET

You should call a vet as soon as possible; these are both situations that will require professional input, particularly if you have never been faced with such a crisis before.

Be aware that your horse is likely to need supportive treatment once it has been released. This may include pain relief, intravenous fluids and appropriate treatment of any other injuries, or in the worst case euthanasia.

HORSE CAUGHT IN A FENCE OR WIRE

FIRST AID FACTS

Around the pastern several important structures lie close to the skin surface, including the joint capsule and the tendon sheath; these structures are therefore particularly vulnerable to injury.

Most accidents result from a horse bolting and running straight through anything that is in its flight path – in this state its adrenalin will be at a high level,so any injuries it has incurred will not hurt much until an hour or so after everything has calmed down. At this point the horse may suddenly go lame.

WHAT TO LOOK FOR

- Your horse in an unusual part of the field, not moving towards you or missing from its paddock, with damage to the fence.

- Check for wire, string/twine or rope tangled around the horse's legs, or any wounds caused by wooden fencing or hedging material.
- If the horse has barged through fencing or a hedge, check for cuts and abrasions, especially in the *axillae* (armpits), the chest and the groin area.
- Check over the head and the eyes thoroughly.

WHAT TO DO

- Injuries tend to become more serious the longer the horse is trapped, as prolonged struggling will only exacerbate any damage already done. Assess if you are able to free the horse on your own, and if you cannot, then call for help immediately and concentrate on keeping the horse calm.

- If there is wire or rope caught around your horse it will need to be cut off. This is easier with two people, as one can distract and calm the horse while the other frees the trapped limb.
- Once the horse is free from its entanglement, check thoroughly for any injuries, even in areas that were not directly entangled.

WHEN TO CALL THE VET

You should call the vet if you are concerned that there is an injury requiring treatment, such as a deep contaminated wound or a long gash, or if you are worried that the wound is in the region of the joint capsule or tendon sheath.

The vet should also be called if your horse is very lame once it has been released, but you cannot see any obvious injuries.

WHAT THE VET MAY DO

Your vet can assess if any injuries to the lower leg have penetrated the joint capsule or tendon sheath, and treat them accordingly; if penetration has occurred, this is an emergency and will require aggressive treatment.

Any wound can be assessed, and anything that requires suturing can be treated accordingly. Pain relief and antibiotics are often required, and tetanus antitoxin may also be given if your horse's vaccinations are not up to date.

(For more information regarding wound care, *see* pages 14–21.)

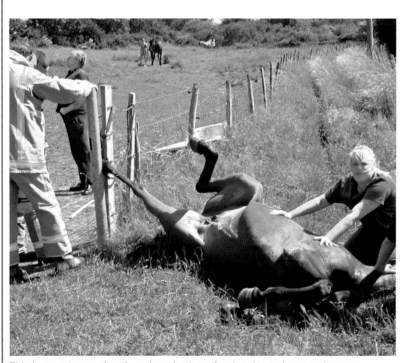

This is an extreme situation where both professional veterinary and rescue services are required. This horse needed an anaesthetic to enable its removal from the fence

128

FALL IN THE TRAILER OR LORRY

FIRST AID FACTS

Most physical injuries from a fall in a trailer or lorry are superficial, and the biggest problem is usually dealing with the phobia that may follow. The greatest risk is of a limb or limbs being trapped under a partition and thereby causing lacerations or fractures of the lower limb(s).

WHAT TO LOOK FOR

- Try and check for any serious cuts and scrapes, or any penetrating injuries.
- Check that the legs are not seriously injured.
- If the horse is trapped, decide if you can lift the partition out of the way on your own, or if cutting equipment will be needed.

WHAT TO DO

- It is vital to keep the horse calm to avoid exacerbating any injuries; you will need help so you can concentrate on the horse while the partition is moved.
- You may find that cotton wool in the horse's ears or a towel as a blindfold helps, but at all times ensure that your safety is taken into consideration.

WHEN TO CALL THE VET

If any of the horse's injuries looks serious – if you suspect a broken leg or a penetrating wound (*see* pages 18 and 40) – or if it is stressed and needs sedating before it can be released, then a vet should be called immediately.

Once the horse has been released, a vet should be called to make sure there are no underlying injuries if it is lame or unsteady on its feet.

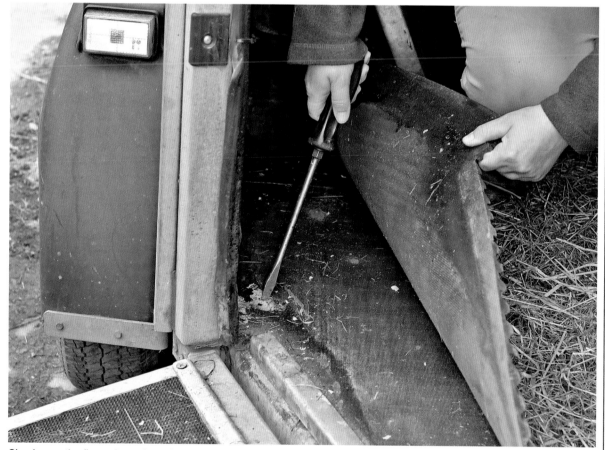

Check over the floor of your horsebox or trailer regularly in order to minimize the risk of your horse putting a foot through it when travelling

INJURIES OUT RIDING

FIRST AID FACTS

Most injuries when out riding are caused by the horse reacting suddenly and unexpectedly to something that frightens him. If you ride out over long distances a small first aid kit is invaluable as providing the means to contain a minor injury, and a mobile phone for summoning help or warning that you will be late.

The majority of injuries received out riding are not serious, and you will be able to hack slowly back to the stable where, if you have rung ahead, help should be available. If an injury looks serious, however, and you think the horse will not be able to walk home, try to ascertain precisely where you are so you can give accurate directions to the vet so they can find you as quickly as possible.

WHAT TO DO

- Often the rider of the injured horse has been unseated, so you should first make sure that they are not hurt. If they have sustained injuries, administer suitable first aid and call for help.
- If you are accompanying the horse and rider who have been injured, make sure you can secure your own horse safely before you investigate the situation further – a loose horse is likely to damage itself, and will risk making an already fragile situation worse.
- Once the injured horse has been caught, run your hands over its legs checking for cuts and grazes as well as foreign bodies – you should pay particular attention to the pastern.
- If you discover a superficial wound, apply basic first aid as described in earlier chapters.
- Decide if the horse (and rider) will be able to walk home, or if treatment or transport is needed from where you are.

WHEN TO CALL THE VET

If you find an injury that requires treatment, for example a laceration or if the horse is very lame, then you will have to decide if, in your opinion, the horse can walk home or not; obviously the distance from home will be a factor in this decision.

If you decide the injury is severe and your horse will not be able to easily walk home, then the vet will need to examine the horse at the site of the accident and administer the necessary treatment before it is transported. If the horse can walk home, arrange for a vet to visit you at your stables.

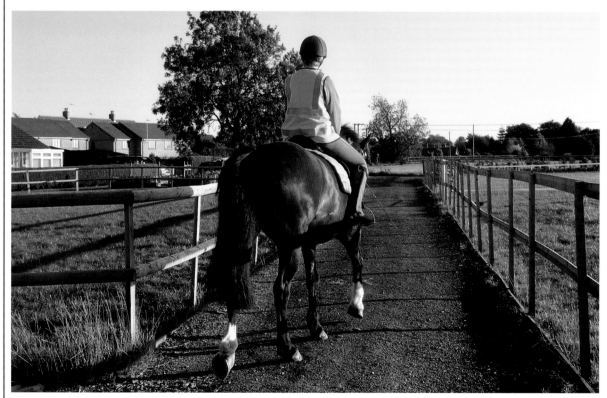

When hacking out, especially alone, make sure you are highly visible and are carrying a mobile phone in case of emergency

HORSE LYING DOWN AND UNABLE TO STAND

FIRST AID FACTS

It is very rare for an apparently completely healthy horse to die suddenly. Remember that a horse can injure you very easily without meaning to, so if it is lying down, always approach it from behind its head and neck, and do not get in between the legs.

WHAT TO LOOK FOR

- Check for breathing and a heartbeat; if you are not sure, touch the corner of the eye gently, as this should make the horse blink. If it is dead there will be no response at all.
- Look at the colour of the gums: if they are anything other than a healthy salmon-pink colour, there is a major problem with the circulation.
- If the gums are normal, check the limbs for injury: they might have become caught in fencing or a rabbit hole.
- Check for other indications of the cause of injury: for example, make sure that the electrical systems are all functioning normally, or look for signs of lightning strike.
- Check any other horses in the field for evidence of injury or illness.

WHAT TO DO

- If there is no obvious injury or illness causing the horse to stay lying down, then encourage it to stand by making plenty of noise.
- If the horse is trying to stand up but is not quite able to make it, then call for assistance to roll the horse on to its other side so it can try and stand using fresh muscles (see Cast Horse, page 126).
- If you are successful in making your horse stand, then you should encourage it to walk slowly around to encourage blood flow to the muscles to help ease any cramps or muscle pain.

WHEN TO CALL THE VET

You should call the vet if your horse shows signs of illness – for example, if the heart rate or breathing is much faster or slower than usual, or the colour of the gums is abnormal – and if there are any signs of obvious injury, for instance to the legs, or if there is asymmetry of the pelvis. In these circumstances do not try and move the horse until the vet has examined it.

If the horse stands, but is wobbly and uncertain once it is standing and unwilling to move, then your vet should examine the horse to make sure there are no injuries, in particular to the pelvis.

PUT YOUR OWN SAFETY FIRST

If you suspect your horse has been electrocuted in the stable you must pay strict attention to your own safety, and ensure there is no risk to yourself before approaching the horse. Find where the main trip switch is for the yard, and turn off all the power before you consider approaching the horse. If you are unsure about your safety, call the emergency services for advice on your situation.

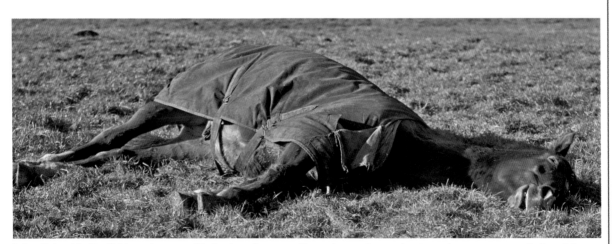

Lying flat out in the field can be normal behaviour; however, if your horse does not get up when you approach, then this may be a sign that there is a problem

COLLAPSING HORSE

FIRST AID FACTS

It is very rare that a horse collapses, but it is usually associated with a catastrophic event such as a heart attack, or the rupture of a major internal organ such as the liver or a major blood vessel.

A winded horse will collapse and appear dead, or be struggling to breathe; as horses are usually winded following a serious fall, there may be other injuries involved. If the horse is simply winded, after a few minutes it will sit up and then eventually stand; some horses will then appear completely normal, while others react strongly to the stress and pain of the incident.

If a horse collapses, do not try and support it or stop it falling: it is much heavier than you, and you will be injured.

WHAT TO DO

- DO NOT APPROACH A THRASHING HORSE OR YOU WILL BE INJURED.
- When the horse is quiet, approach carefully towards its back, avoiding its legs, and talking to it all the time so it knows where you are, even though it can't see you.
- Check for a pulse, for breathing, and if you are still in doubt, check the blink (palpebral) reflex.
- If there is a pulse and the horse blinks, check the colour of the gums; you should also check for dehydration or signs of trauma.

- If the horse is distressed, use a sweatshirt as a blindfold and keep talking and stroking it to keep it calm.
- Check for any injuries, especially to the limbs. Be very careful while you do this, as you can very easily be injured: if possible try to lean over the body to examine the legs – do not get in between them.
- Keep the horse as warm as possible until help arrives: use rugs where you can, or coats if necessary.
- If the horse is able to sit up but not stand, then you can offer some water.

WHEN TO CALL THE VET

Once you have established the horse is still alive you should call a vet to check it over, even if it has got up and appears to have recovered. If a winded horse has not stood up within 3 to 5 minutes, you should call for veterinary assistance.

TOP TIP

If a horse has collapsed and is not moving, you can find out if it is still alive by touching the corner of the eye: the horse should blink, and if it does not, it is dead. This is called the palpebral, or 'blink reflex'.

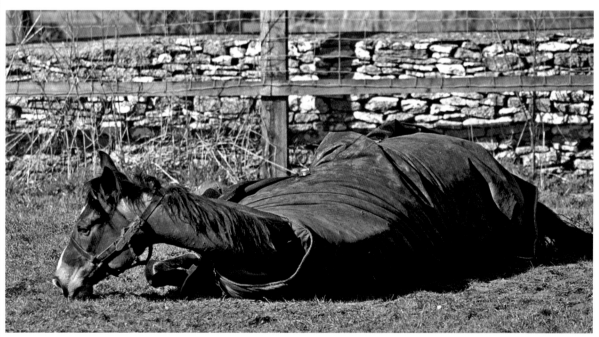

When a horse is down and struggling, be very careful how you approach it; make sure you approach from its back, talking to it at all times, and keeping out of range of its legs

UNEXPECTED FOALING

Unexpected pregnancy is a common complication when acquiring a new mare, especially from auctions and sales. However, although a new foal might be a huge surprise to you, the majority of mares experience very few complications when giving birth.

DISCOVERING A FOAL

FIRST AID FACTS

Mares prefer privacy when foaling, and can stop labour for prolonged periods if they feel threatened, so unless you think your mare is having difficulties try and keep quiet and out of sight – this is why most studs have CCTV to monitor the foaling box.

It is very important that the placenta is passed in one piece within about four hours of the foal's birth: a retained placenta can pose serious health risks for the mare, as complications can develop within a matter of hours.

It is also vital that a foal suckles within the first few hours of life, as the mare produces special milk (**colostrum**) in the first twelve hours of the foal's life: this first milk has a very high level of antibodies which protect the foal against common infections.

WHAT TO LOOK FOR

- Check the mare for any signs of pain (sweating, fast pulse or rapid breathing), check the vulva to make sure that there is not a large amount of blood present, and check that she has milk in her udder. Many mares run milk shortly before and after giving birth. If the mare's udder feels hot, hard or painful to the touch she may have mastitis (see p.80), which will need rapid treatment from the vet.
- Check the placenta – this should be a pink/red colour and velvety in texture, and T- or Y-shaped (*see* page 135). It is very important that you check the placenta thoroughly to ensure it has all been passed, as any

---

THE PROPERTIES OF COLOSTRUM

During the first 12 hours of a foal's life the gut has a special ability to absorb antibodies from its mother's milk; this heightened permeability only lasts for these 12 hours, after which the gut will only absorb nutrients and not antibodies. As a result of this, the composition of the mare's colostrum changes after these first few hours after birth, decreasing in quality until it has the composition of normal milk after two to three days. If your mare is 'running milk' before she is due to foal, it is beneficial to the foal to collect this milk and store it hygienically until it is born, and then use this milk as the first feed.

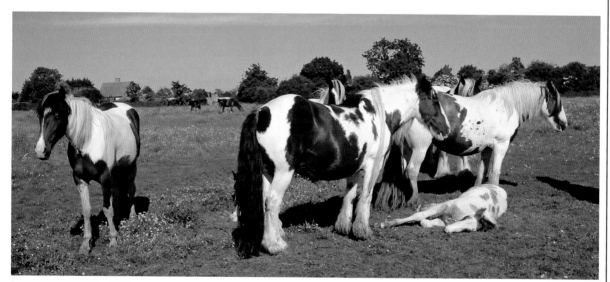

Mares and foals in a field

tissue that is retained can cause very serious illness very quickly. A normal placenta should have a tear in one end where the foal has come through, but otherwise should be largely intact.

- Check the foal – it should be able to stand and suckle within one to two hours of birth (colts sometimes take longer than fillies to do this). Check the umbilical cord is clean and dry, and that there is no swelling in this area; also check in the groin for swellings.

WHAT TO DO
- If the foal is struggling to find the udder, some gentle direction and guidance to help it fasten on to the teat for the first time can stimulate it into greater effort.
- Dip or treat the umbilical stump with disinfectant to reduce the risk of infection entering the body here.

WHEN TO CALL THE VET
If this is your first experience of a foal it is a good idea to contact your vet for advice, and ideally arrange a check-over for mum and baby. However, if you notice any of the following symptoms, veterinary advice is urgently needed:
- If the mare appears distressed or in pain, or is showing signs of colic.
- If there appears to be excessive

bleeding or tissue protruding from the vulva – this may mean either a prolapse of the uterus or vagina, or be a sign of internal damage.
- If you are worried about the condition of the mare's udder or the amount of milk she has.
- If you are not sure that the entire placenta has been passed.
- If the mare is showing signs of laminitis (an uncommon complication following birth).
- If the foal has been unable to stand or suckle milk.
- If there is milk coming down the foal's nose: this may indicate a cleft palate.
- If the foal was bright and active, but becomes subdued over the first 24 hours of life: this is an emergency as neonatal foals are very susceptible to a range of serious conditions.
- If the foal's abdomen becomes very bloated, or you have not seen it pass the **meconium** (first faeces).
- If there are any swellings on the foal, for example between the back legs, under the abdomen, or over any of the joints.

WHAT THE VET MAY DO
Post-foaling colic in the mare is potentially very serious, as there is a greatly increased risk of a twist in the gut because of the space that

has suddenly become available in the abdomen. Your vet will therefore check your mare very carefully, and if they have any cause for concern, may suggest referral to a hospital where a close, continuous watch can be kept on the mare for any development in her condition.

Laminitis following foaling is also very serious, as it is often caused by a build-up of toxins in the body, often as a result of the placenta not being fully passed. Antibiotics in combination with treatment to clean the uterus may be used in conjunction with the standard treatment for laminitis. An oxytocin drip in conjunction with antibiotics will be used if a retained placenta is suspected.

Any tears in the vagina or vulva should be repaired as quickly as possible to promote healthy healing. Poor healing or scarring in this area can affect the shape and structure of the vagina, leading to conditions such as pooling of urine in the vagina, or faecal contamination of the vagina, with consequences for uterine health and future fertility.

Sometimes a foal may have abnormal tendons, in that they are either too tight (congenital contracted tendons) or too loose (flexor tendon laxity). Either of these problems must be addressed quickly to give the foal a chance of survival. Depending on the degree of severity of the problem, splints, casts or corrective shoeing may be necessary.

A ruptured bladder is not uncommon in foals; it is caused by the trauma of birth. This condition requires urgent surgical correction or the foal will rapidly become toxic and die.

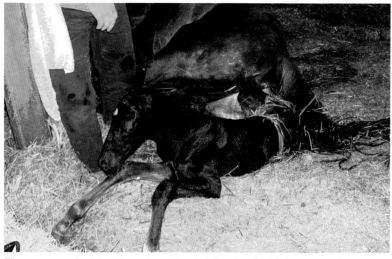

The mare remains lying down immediately following the birth to allow all the blood in the placenta to circulate into the foal

DISCOVERING YOUR MARE FOALING

Try not to worry, as most mares will give birth on their own. You should also try to watch from a discrete distance, as even the most trusting mare may be upset by intrusions during the birth process.

WHAT TO LOOK FOR

- Most mares will lie down in the final stages of labour; a milky white sac should appear from the vulva, which will be followed by a pair of feet, the head and then the rest of the body. The foal should break through this sac on its own.
- Once the foal has been delivered, the mare may remain lying down for a few minutes: this allows as much blood as possible to be retained in the foal's body before the umbilical cord is ruptured by the mare standing up. It is very important not to disturb the mare at this stage, as standing up too quickly can rupture the umbilical cord too early and possibly damage the placenta or the uterus lining.

WHAT TO DO

- If you see your mare go into labour, put a tail bandage on to help keep the area clean and prevent contamination during this sensitive time.

THE THREE STAGES OF LABOUR

Labour has three stages. The first stage is when uterine contractions begin, which helps position the foal correctly for birth. The mare will often be restless and will twitch her tail, and may yawn or lie down repeatedly. The end of the first stage is when the sac surrounding the foal breaks.

The second stage starts as the foal moves into the birth canal, abdominal straining starts, and the mare will lie down on her side until the foal is born. This stage should take about 15 minutes; if it lasts longer than an hour, veterinary assistance is required. If the foal is born normally the mare will stay lying down for up to 10 minutes to allow all of the foal's blood which is still in the placenta to reach the foal. When the mare stands up the umbilical cord will be broken.

The third stage is the expulsion of the placenta, which normally happens between one and two hours following birth. If this does not happen, or if, on inspection, there appears to be part of the placenta missing, veterinary advice should be sought immediately as this has the potential to make the mare very ill.

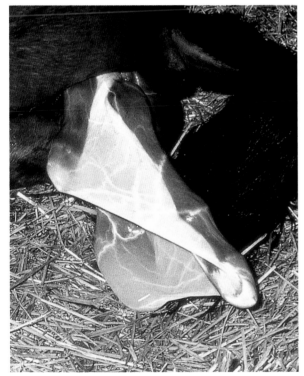

Second stage labour: in a normal birth you will see a white sac emerge with the two front hooves and the foal's nose showing within it

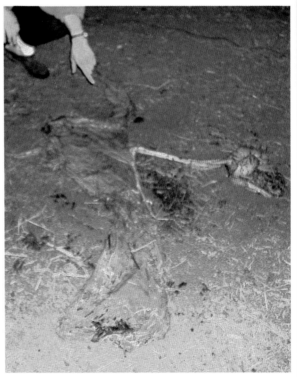

Check the placenta thoroughly to make sure none has been left behind

- You should intervene if the foal has been delivered but has not broken through the bag: simply clear the membranes from over the foal's nose, and clear any mucus from the nose and upper part of the throat. A brisk rub on the chest is usually adequate to stimulate the foal's breathing.
- Once the foal has been born for about 10 minutes, if the mare has not already stood up, the foal can be moved towards her head to encourage her mothering instincts and to avoid injury to the foal as she gets to her feet.

WHEN TO CALL THE VET

- If the second stage of labour is taking more than 45 minutes.
- If the bag that appears at the vulva is red and velvety in appearance, rather than milky and smooth.
- If the foal's legs do not appear together, or if the head does not quickly follow the legs.

WHAT THE VET MAY DO

The vet may be able to assist the mare in giving birth to the foal by rearranging the position of the foal in the uterus if the presentation is not normal, for example by bringing a leg forwards if both front legs are not in the birth canal. If the amniotic sac is too thick for the foal to rupture on its own, then this can be broken (breaking the waters) to allow labour to progress.

If the position of the foal cannot be corrected, then a caesarean section may be suggested. However, this is a high risk procedure for both mare and foal, and requires a general anaesthetic, so it will only be suggested if there is no alternative.

136

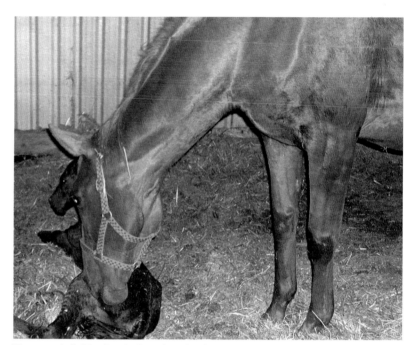

The mare is licking her foal to clean it and to stimulate it to stand and suckle

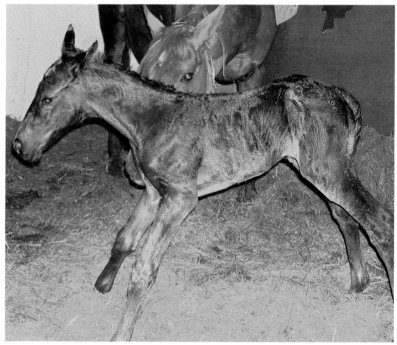

The foal should stand and suckle within an hour of birth

SNAKE BITE

FIRST AID FACTS

Snakes are very sensitive to vibrations and usually get out of the way when they feel a larger animal approaching. Not all snake bites, even from venomous snakes, contain venom, as sometimes the snake will give a warning bite first.

Horses are more sensitive to snake venom than most other mammals, but the size of a horse means that the venom is unlikely to be sufficient to cause death. The severity of the bite's effect depends on the type of snake and where on the horse's body the bite has been inflicted: thus some snakes are more venomous than others, while bites to the face and neck are more serious than bites to the extremities or the body.

The type of snake that could threaten your horse depends on your location, so it is well worth getting to know the snakes in your area and learning to recognize the venomous and non-venomous 'locals'.

WHAT TO LOOK FOR

- Most bites occur on the muzzle because they are inflicted while the horse is grazing.
- The area immediately surrounding the bite will start to swell rapidly, although you should still be able to identify the puncture marks made by the fangs.
- If the bite is on the muzzle the swelling can be severe enough to block the nostrils.
- Intense pain reaction, muscle weakness and shock can rapidly develop following a venomous bite.

WHAT TO DO

- If your horse is bitten when you are out riding, try and calm it down as quickly as possible, because a rapid heart rate caused by exercise or excitement can speed the spread of the venom within the horse's body.
- Try and back your horse slowly away from the snake to prevent a second bite, and don't let your horse put its face down to investigate either, as the muzzle is a sensitive area to be bitten.
- In areas where extremely venomous snakes are found, experienced horse riders or ranchers carry two 6in cut-offs of garden hose, which can be inserted into the nostrils to prevent complete obstruction of the airways by swelling. If you are unfamiliar with this technique, seek advice from experienced locals.
- If the bite is on a lower limb, then apply pressure above the bite to reduce the spread of the venom in the body. This tourniquet should be tight enough to restrict blood flow in the veins and lymphatics, but not the arteries; a broad band such as a bandage, handkerchief or clothing should be used as the tourniquet to minimize the damage caused to underlying tissues.
- Walk you horse slowly back to your yard, or if possible use a trailer as transport, because reducing the amount of movement the horse needs to do will minimize the spread of the venom within the body.
- DO NOT cut the wound open, OR try and suck the venom from the wound, OR apply hot or cold compresses, as these have all been shown to exacerbate the situation.

OTHER VENOMOUS CREATURES

Venomous snakes are not the only cause of poisonous bites: depending on your geographical location there may also be a risk from other reptiles, spiders or scorpions. Treatment for bites from these creatures is symptomatic, along the same lines as for a snake bite; anti-venom may also be available if you are able to accurately identify what creature bit your horse.

WHEN TO CALL THE VET

You should call your vet as soon as possible after you realize your horse as been bitten, as the faster treatment can be initiated, the better the prognosis will be for a good recovery.

WHAT THE VET MAY DO

Treatment should cover three major points:

1. Reducing the spread of the venom in the horse's body: you will have begun this process by applying a tourniquet where possible, and by keeping your horse calm and restricting its movement.
2. Counteracting the effects of the venom with suitable anti-venom if appropriate. The use of suitable anti-venom will depend on you being able to accurately identify the snake that bit your horse. You should also be aware that there is a risk of your horse developing anaphylaxis in response to the anti-venom; some vets will give adrenalin (epinephrine) at the same time as the anti-venom to counter this effect.
3. Maintaining respiratory and cardiovascular function; the amount of treatment required will depend on the severity of the bite and the type of snake involved. Pain relief and antibiotics are always required, steroids may be given if shock is developing, and in severe cases intravenous fluids will also be given to support the circulation.

Once the initial reaction to the bite has resolved there will be tissue damage, and this will need to be treated as any other open wound, under direction of your vet.

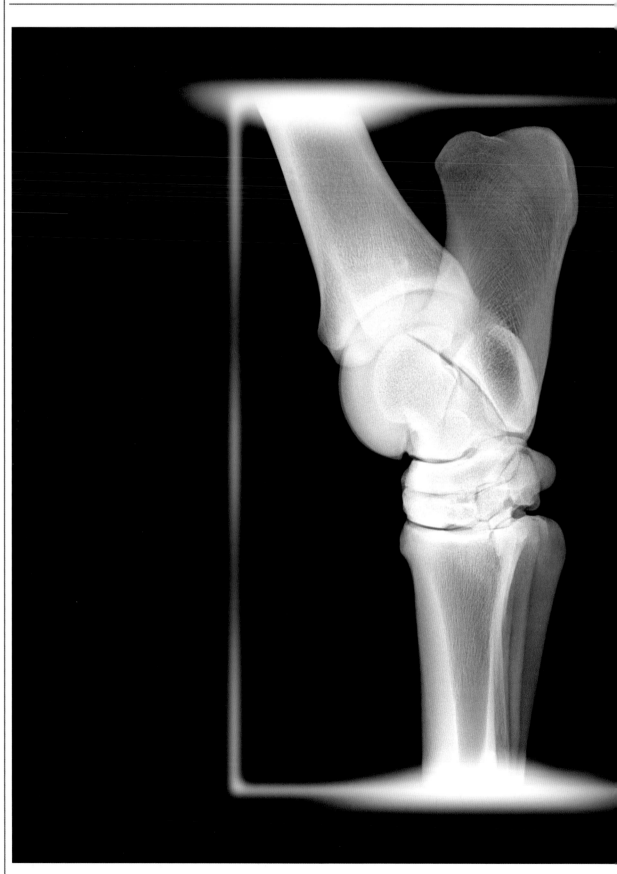

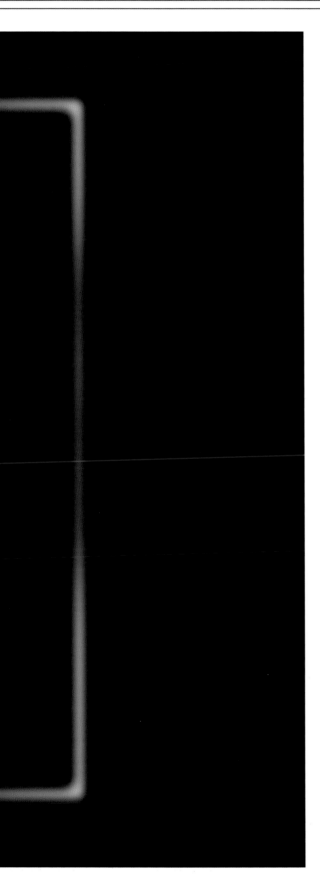

SECTION 4
DIAGNOSTIC PROCEDURES AND TREATMENTS

This section explains some of the most commonly used diagnostic techniques used by your vet, when and why they are used, the useful information which can be learnt from them, and how the information provided can benefit your horse and influence the treatment plan.

TECHNICAL INVESTIGATIONS

ULTRASOUND

Ultrasound is a very useful technique which is being used in many different ways as technology develops. Ultrasound images are produced by low-level soundwaves being emitted from a head which alternates between sending and receiving signals. The signal detected depends on the underlying tissues, as each tissue type reflects the signal differently. Dense tissue reflects the signal strongly and shows up white, and white fluid shows up as black because it absorbs the signal. This is why a foetus shows clearly as a skeleton floating in a sack, because the limbs reflect strongly while the fluid absorbs the signal.

The two most common areas for which ultrasound is used are the lower limbs, to look at tendon and ligament structure, and the reproductive tract, to look at the ovaries to asses the optimum moment to inseminate, and at the uterus to check for its health and pregnancy status, and in order to diagnose the presence of twins.

Depending on the ability of the person using the scanner, as well as the scope of the machine, ultrasound can also be used to visualize the abdomen – most commonly in foals to help diagnose a ruptured bladder, but increasingly in horses referred for surgical colic because it allows visualization of the abnormalities of the abdomen prior to surgery, thereby allowing more accurate planning of the surgery.

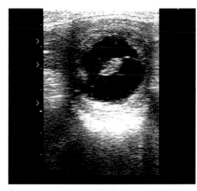

Pregnancy diagnosis is a common use of ultrasound equipment, this is the typical image produced by a foetus in the first month of pregnancy; the dark area is the amniotic fluid in which the foetus is floating

X-RAYS

Despite the advent of more technologically advanced imaging techniques, x-rays remain a very useful part of the diagnostic tool kit. The x-ray machines are generally portable, and will rapidly produce easily interpreted images, at least in the case of many major disorders; the more modern techniques come into play with conditions that are subtle and difficult to diagnose by x-ray.

X-ray machines work in the following way: they use electricity to produce x-rays, high-energy radioactive waves that are channelled through the object to be imaged on to an x-ray. The image is produced on light-sensitive film as a result of the x-rays bombarding the special lining of the cassette to produce tiny particles of light. This light causes the film to react, and the more light, the greater the reaction. Once the film is processed, the areas with the greatest reaction show up as dark areas, while the areas with the least reaction show as white areas. Soft tissue does not stop the x-rays, so these areas show up as either dark or grey areas, depending on the density of the tissue, while bone stops x-rays so will show as white – cracks in the bone will be visible as dark lines.

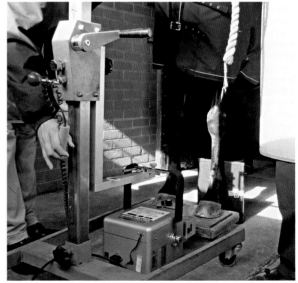

Foot x-rays being taken; note the protective lead apron being worn by the vet

Digital x-rays are now revolutionizing the use of x-ray machines, because the image can be manipulated as if greater or smaller amounts of x-rays have passed through the object. This reduces the number of times a patient has to be exposed to the radiation, and allows a greater number of diagnoses to be made from a single image.

NUCLEAR SCINTIGRAPHY

This is an imaging technique used to look for subtle lesions that have not shown up using other techniques. The horse must be admitted to a veterinary hospital for this technique because the horse itself, and its urine and faeces, will be radioactive immediately after this procedure has been performed.

The horse is injected with a harmless radioactive isotope, *Technicium 99*, which remains in the blood but has an affinity for bone. After a rest period to allow the isotope to spread throughout the body, the horse is moved to a special imaging screen and a gamma camera is used to measure the radioactive particles being emitted by the horse. This is a very painstaking procedure, as each position that the camera is moved to requires the horse to remain absolutely stationary for approximately two minutes with a strange object hovering over its body!

The images produced are primarily of the skeleton, although if a longer rest period is used some facilities are able to image soft tissue lesions. Areas of inflammation show as a stronger colour (usually red); these are most commonly stress fractures.
There are two different levels of pre-purchase examination that you can request a vet to perform

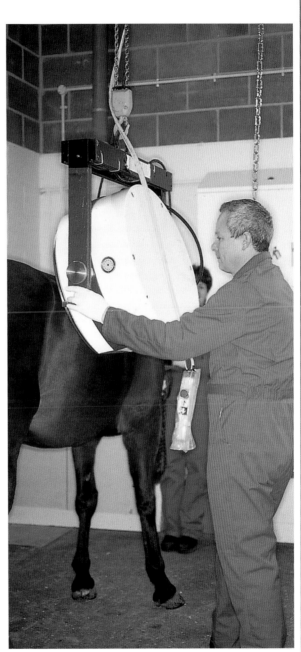

This large camera is reading the radioactive emissions from the horse's pelvis

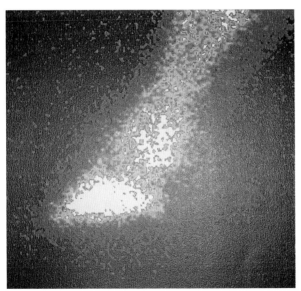

The different colours on this scan relate to different intensities of radioactivity; red areas show higher levels of activity caused by increased blood flow due to inflammation

DIAGNOSTIC TESTS

MEDICATING JOINTS

This technique is used following diagnosis of a problem in a specific joint, for example arthritis. The medication is injected in the same manner as described for joint blocks. Medicating the joints is usually aimed at either preventing further damage to the cartilage, or preventing the formation of further new arthritic bone (usually using hyularonic acid), or at relieving pain and inflammation (usually using steroids).

As with joint blocks, there is a risk of contamination causing an infection in the joint, so some vets use a low dose of antibiotic at the same time – particularly when steroids are injected – to reduce this risk.

BLOOD TESTS

Blood tests can be divided into three areas: haematology, biochemistry and endocrinology.

Haematology involves counting the number of red blood cells, and the number and type of white blood cells, which gives a picture of events in the body. This can indicate the type of inflammation – whether infectious or allergic, and whether a viral infection is involved – and can give a timescale to the condition by the number, size and shape of different types of cell.

Biochemistry is a measurement of the enzymes released by the organs in the body in response to stress, disease or injury. The main markers used are related to liver, kidney or muscle. The levels of these markers need to be considered in comparison with the haematology and the symptoms. Interpretation of the results so as to give a meaningful diagnosis takes considerable skill.

Endocrinology is a measurement of the hormones in the bloodstream; it is usually part of a further investigation, for example to confirm a metabolic disorder such as Cushings. It can be used as a pregnancy diagnosis in mares that are either too small or are temperamentally unsuitable for rectal examination.

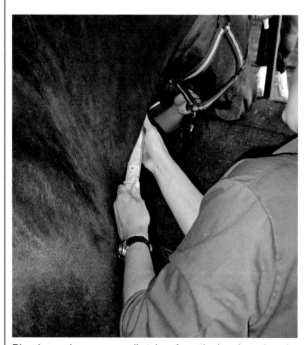
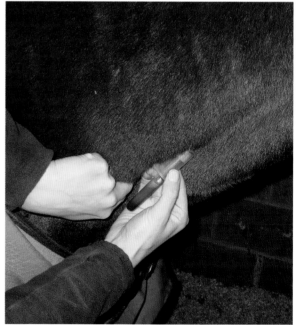

Blood samples are normally taken from the jugular vein using either a needle and syringe or directly into the storage tubes, which contain anticoagulents

NERVE AND JOINT BLOCKS

This technique is used to locate the source of pain, particularly in stubborn lameness cases. Local anaesthetic is injected either directly into a joint capsule (if arthritis is suspected – usually following a positive reaction to a flexion test) or directly over a nerve.

Nerve blocks can be a very long drawn-out procedure, depending on the cause of the lameness and its position in the leg. There is a paired nerve supply to the foot, which follows a symmetrical pattern down the leg and is close to the surface at several points. These points are used to inject the local anaesthetic, starting at the lowest point of the leg, usually the back of the pastern: small amounts are injected over the nerve and then, following a wait to allow the local anaesthetic to work, the horse is trotted up and an assessment is made of the effect on the lameness.

Depending on the degree of improvement or otherwise of the lameness, further nerve blocks are gradually performed higher up the leg until a point is found where the lameness is alleviated. Usually nerve blocks above the knee or hock are only performed at a referral centre, because they are technically very difficult. The cause of the lameness is usually found between the block that improved the lameness, and the block performed previously.

Joint blocks require a high degree of asepsis, so the area over the joint will be clipped and then scrubbed up as if for surgery, the vet will then put on sterile gloves before putting a needle through the skin into the joint. This is a very demanding technique, and the horse may require restraint – sedation or a twitch – to allow it to be performed safely and effectively. There is a small risk of infection developing in the joint following this technique, so it is important that your horse is closely monitored for 48 hours afterwards.

Joints that are painful and causing lameness will be numbed by the local anaesthetic, and the lameness should improve significantly; if this is the case your vet may opt to inject medication into the joint to improve the condition and control pain on a long-term basis.

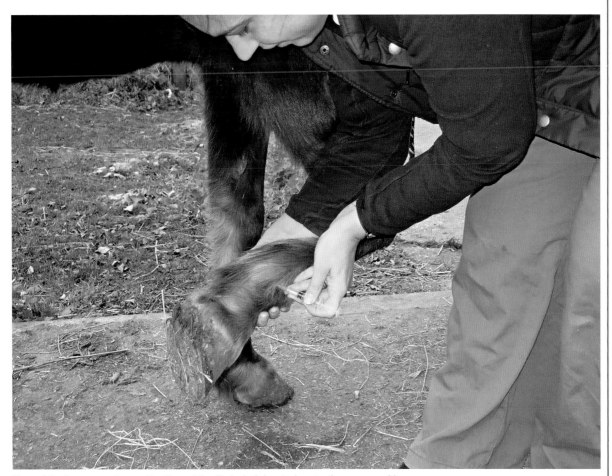

Nerve blocks cause desensitization of the limb, helping to locate the source of lameness

PRE-PURCHASE EXAMINATION

Performed by the vet, on your behalf: a *two-stage vetting*, and a *five-stage vetting*. The *two-stage vetting* is a very basic examination consisting of the following tests:

Stage 1 A full physical examination that includes listening to the heart, lungs and gut, an ophthalmic examination, and manual palpation of the whole body to check for lumps, bumps, swellings or signs of pain, injury or illness – this includes checking for sarcoids. Assuming that no abnormalities are found in the course of this stage, the vet will proceed to the second stage: soundness evaluation.

Stage 2 Soundness evaluation – in fact evaluating the horse for signs of lameness. This involves a walk- and trot-up, followed by flexion tests on all four limbs.

The *five-stage vetting* includes the two-stage vetting, plus the following three stages:

Stage 3 The vet assesses the horse at exercise, either ridden or lunged: he will see the horse perform its three basic paces on both reins, and will then ask for the horse to be exerted until it is puffing. This allows an evaluation of the heart and lungs under stress, and should show up any abnormal noise, gait or respiratory problem.

Stage 4 Involves an evaluation of the horse's recovery following exercise; a further physical examination, including checking the teeth; and an inspection of the horse's available documentation (passports should always be to hand) in order to confirm the identity of the horse being presented for examination; the vet will also take a blood sample, the results of which will reveal whether the horse has been given unauthorized drugs that would mask unsoundness (and see below).

Stage 5 A re-examination for lameness, which involves repeating all the trotting and flexion tests, as well as pushing the horse in hand in a small circle on each rein, and backwards, in order to check for physical problems that might have been exacerbated by the earlier exercise. A final examination of the legs and chest will be made.

With both the two-stage and the five-stage examinations it is recommended that the buyer should be present. This enables them to see exactly what the vet is doing, and for the vet to discuss anything relevant with them at the time, particularly if the horse is going to fail the examination; it therefore also reduces the potential for dispute should there be any problems in the future.

The blood sample which is taken at the time of the vetting is normally stored for six months after the vetting;

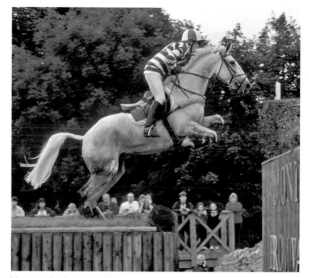

You can't always tell if a horse has a medical problem just by looking at it: a professional opinion can be useful when making an expensive purchase

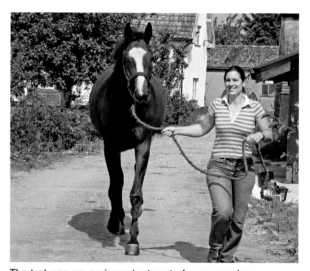

The trot-ups are an important part of a pre-purchase examination

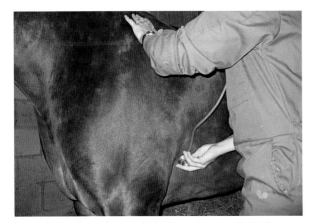

Careful attention will be paid to the noises made by the heart and lungs at several stages of the examination

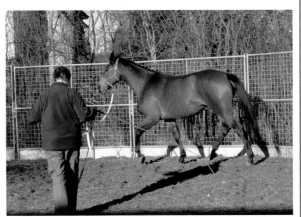

Lungeing may be used in stage 3 if a suitable rider is not available, or if the horse is not broken to saddle

the purpose of this sample is so that checks can be made for medication that the horse may have been given, which would have affected its performance on the day of the vetting. The sample can be tested at any time if, for example, the horse suddenly goes lame or has a violent change in personality.

Further examinations can be performed depending on the value and the use of the horse; for example, high performance show jumpers that are being sold on to continue competing may have x-rays taken of the major joints (for example, the hocks or fetlocks): this is at the expense of the buyer. If a problem is highlighted during the vetting, then further investigation may be suggested by the vet before they can recommend that the buyer continues with the purchase.

Many insurance companies require a pre-purchase certificate before starting a policy. A similar examination can be undertaken for a horse that is already in your possession if the insurance company requires it; again, this would be at the owner's expense.

Finally, a pre-purchase examination is not a guarantee of a horse's soundness or health: it is a snapshot of the horse at the time of the examination. The examination is very thorough and often highlights issues that even the sellers were not aware of, and while the examination is only relating to the health of the horse, many vets will discuss the horse in a great deal more detail, as well as its suitability for the job intended for it.

FLEXION TESTS

Flexion tests are performed usually as part of a lameness investigation, or as part of a five-stage vetting. The horse is held at the head by the person who will trot it up in hand in the second part of the test: thus the vet will hold the leg to be tested at full flexion for a full minute, and as soon as this minute is up, the horse is led away straight into a trot in a straight line. In this test it is the first few paces that are the most important.

The aim of the flexion test is to stretch the joints in the limb as fully as possible in order to exacerbate any discomfort already present. It is most effective at highlighting problems in the lower joints – namely the fetlock and the knee/hock – although with some skill the higher joints can also be stretched. The first few trot paces are the most important because any mild discomfort caused by the flexion will show up with movement, and the horse will trot lame.

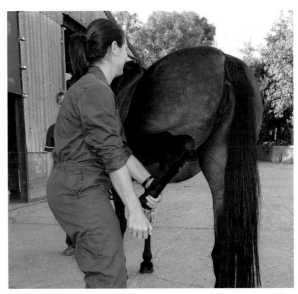

The vet will hold the leg to be tested at full flexion for a full minute

CORRECTIVE TREATMENTS

PHYSIOTHERAPY

Physiotherapy involves a combination of massage, manipulations and stretches to allow muscles to move correctly. This process is useful to aid recovery following a fall or other injury which has caused chronic lameness because the balance of the body has been upset: the resulting tension in muscles can cause further lameness or poor performance. Physiotherapy is also used in performance horses to aid recovery following strenuous exercise, such as between the stages of a three-day event.

Exercises should only be carried out following guidance and regular monitoring by either a vet or a qualified and registered equine physiotherapist, as both have undergone extensive training in anatomy and will ensure that the lameness or focus of pain is correctly identified so that suitable and effective exercises can be carried out. Most courses of treatment, following initial assessment, involve careful manual examination and massage to ease muscles before stretches are performed; the responses and degree of movement will be monitored, and follow-up visits will be arranged to ensure that progress is being made.

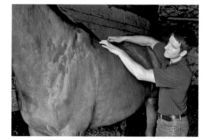

Physiotherapy should be performed by qualified individuals

CORRECTIVE FARRIERY

Corrective farriery has a very broad range of uses, from correcting tendon deformities in foals to supporting laminitis cases in older ponies. Always check that your farrier is registered with the Honourable Company of Farriers before treatment – or even normal shoeing – is carried out.

If your horse is being treated for an abnormal foot shape or other foot condition it is useful to take photos before, during and after treatment to assess the change: feet are slow-growing, and you may not appreciate any real change because you see them on a daily basis.

Most farriers performing corrective farriery will be doing so in conjunction with, and usually at the request of, a vet. Usually x-rays are taken of the feet from several angles before treatment begins to allow a three-dimensional view of the inside of the foot, and the exact position of the pedal bone in relation to the hoof capsule. Different materials to standard metal shoes may be used, as well as dietary supplements to encourage rapid healthy hoof growth to speed up the rate of correction (normal growth is approximately 1cm (½in) per month).

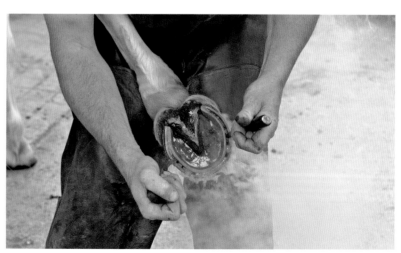

A good farrier can be hard to find

COMPLIMENTARY THERAPIES

ACUPUNCTURE

Acupuncture in animals follows the same principle as acupuncture in humans, that being the use of very fine needles to stimulate nerves at certain points along specific meridians: this can help to control chronic pain. Acupuncture is usually used in animals that have not responded to the standard medical treatments (such as non-steroidal anti-inflammatories), and is used as a treatment of last resort. The effects vary between animals: in some the improvements are rapid and profound, leading to an apparent complete loss of pain and return to normal function; in others this response is slower, or less complete; and some do not respond at all.

There are a number of veterinary surgeons who are qualified and experienced at performing acupuncture, or who work in conjunction with an acupuncturist who has diversified from the practice of standard acupuncture.

Acupuncture can be a very effective treatment, but always discuss the suitability of your horse for this procedure before undertaking what can be a long and expensive course of action, and one that may be ultimately frustrating if your horse is not suitable for treatment.

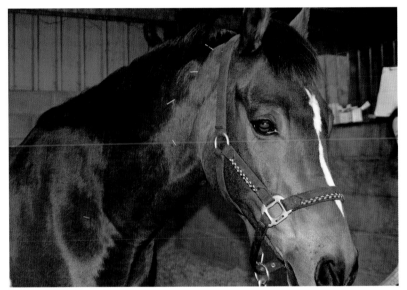

Acupuncture is very well tolerated in the majority of horses; most will relax completely during a treatment, almost appearing to be in a trance

HOMOEOPATHY

Homoeopathy is the use of herbs and very small concentrations of substances to heal the body; its use is very controversial as there is currently little scientific evidence to support its effectiveness. However, many people have reported a very positive response to homoeopathic treatment both in themselves and their animals (in which the placebo effect is harder to use as a reason for effectiveness).

A handful of veterinary surgeons already qualified through the standard universities, and members of the regulatory body (RCVS), have gone on to further study and use homoeopathy in unison with standard veterinary medicine – while some others use homoeopathy alone. If you are interested in this line of approach to treat a condition your horse is suffering from, it is important to discuss your plans with your vet because some homoeopathic treatments contain elements (for example, St John's Wort) that affect the way veterinary drugs are absorbed, and can cause unexpected side effects.

MAINTAINING HEALTH

BOX REST

This is one of the prescriptions that the horse owner most dreads, particularly if the box rest is to be prolonged following serious injury or illness. Trying to balance the restriction in exercise necessary to allow a full recovery with a bored and fretful horse can be extremely stressful. It is simply not possible to box rest some horses because of their tendency to box walk, weave or indulge in some other stable vice, which means they do not rest completely and so slow down the healing process. The methods used to alleviate the stress and boredom of box rest and keep both you and your horse sane need to be discussed with your vet so that the chances of exacerbating the condition are minimized. Here are some suggestions to help the time pass more quickly:

1   Encourage the horse to forage for food – in a wild environment most of a horse's time is spent looking for, and eating, high fibre forage, so try and replicate this in the stable (it may be a bit messy) as a horse can clear its daily allowance from a haynet in one to two hours, and then has nothing to do until your next visit. You can try spreading the hay around the edge of the stable, or using a special hay 'bag' which only has a small window for eating through to slow your horse down. You can also leave surprises such as carrots around the stable to encourage foraging.

2   Have a friend nearby – horses are sociable creatures and often have a best friend, so if possible try and give the friends some time together so your horse is not in on his own all day, but has someone to 'talk to'. This will also help him to feel less vulnerable, because then at least some of the 'herd' is about.

3   Try and keep other horses within eyesight so that your horse does not feel abandoned by the rest of the 'herd'.

4   Give him 'toys' to play with – for example, food balls which can be kicked around the stable and slowly release food: this encourages interaction and foraging behaviour, but the food is released only slowly. The down side is that not all horses have the patience to play with these, and some simply ignore them from the start.

5   Provide a playpen – a small, stable-sized pen which allows for a change of scenery, or allows your horse to be near friends. This is usually only possible if your horse has respect for electric fencing, or if you have an area between paddocks that is normally gated already.

6   Hang up some 'mirrors' – polished steel acts as a safe mirror, giving your horse something moving to look at (itself!) and the impression of having company.

7   Provide music – having the radio on gives a level of background noise that herd animals find reassuring: in the wild there is usually only total silence just before a predator appears over the horizon.

8   Use your imagination and be guided by your horse!

Be prepared for an 'explosion', particularly when you are mucking out and your horse sees its chance to escape, or when you first start leading out in hand. Being prepared for this will prevent your horse escaping and undoing all the good that box rest had achieved so far!

Discuss any changes you are making with your vet first to make sure they will not adversely affect the condition for which your horse is being rested!

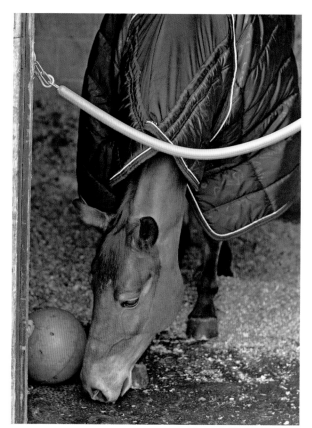

Using a feed ball can stimulate your horse to forage, which helps to pass the time during box rest

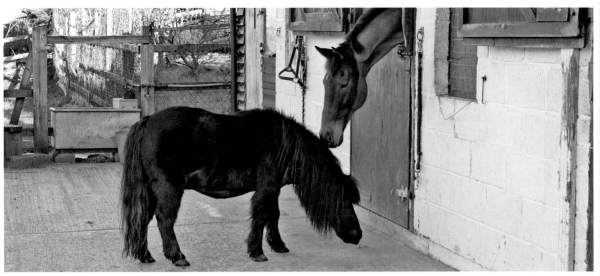

Having a friend close to hand will help keep your horse calm during box rest

VACCINATIONS

Vaccinations are important in maintaining the health of your horse and protecting it from a range of diseases. They work by showing the immune system a 'safe' version of the infectious disease (usually a killed version of a virus, or a modified version which does not cause disease) so that the body learns to recognize the disease and produces antibodies against it, but it does not cause illness. The effectiveness of any vaccine varies, depending on how close an imitation to the real thing it can be, and whether the infectious agent is mutating (changing) – for example, developing into a new strain of equine influenza.

There are a number of different conditions which can be vaccinated against, and it is best to speak to your vet to find out what is recommended in your region. The following four conditions are the most common equine diseases which are vaccinated against.

1   *Tetanus* – If you vaccinate for nothing else, this is a 'must': the infectious agent *Clostridium tetani* is present in the soil and normally introduced through puncture wounds where bacteria grow rapidly in the anaerobic environment, producing the tetanus toxin. Tetanus is thankfully very rare in modern conditions; where it is diagnosed there is rarely an obvious wound to blame it on – which increases the importance of vaccination, as the risk is not easily identifiable, as it is with other diseases. An initial vaccination course for tetanus is generally two injections two or three weeks apart followed by regular boosters (timing will vary with local licensing depending on the local risk).

2   *Equine influenza* – This is the second most common vaccine used. Equine influenza – 'flu – is primarily spread by close contact with infected horses. The protection your horse receives from one injection can last up to 15 months depending on the brand, but during this period the strength of the protection gradually decreases. Some equine organizations have a maximum period between boosters; for example, the Jockey Club (UK) specifies that booster vaccination should be within 365 days, while the FEI requires 'flu booster vaccination every six months. While 'flu, unlike tetanus, is not usually fatal (with the exception of the very young or very old horses), it can be severely debilitating and full recovery can be prolonged. An initial vaccination course for 'flu (often given in combination with tetanus) is two injections 4–6 weeks apart followed by a third injection 5–6 months after the second injection; this leads on to annual boosters.

3   *Equine herpes* – This is associated with both respiratory and reproductive problems, especially in youngstock. It is often required at high levels of competition, or in very large livery yards. It requires a booster every six months, so it is often given in conjunction with the 'flu boosters required according to FEI rules.

4   *Strangles* – Vaccines against this condition are still variable in their efficiency: in some countries an intramuscular vaccine is available, although it is of questionable efficacy; in other countries a vaccine has been developed that is given into the upper lip – although this, too, is still in its early stages, and efficacy has yet to be fully proved. However, it is useful in the face of an outbreak of the disease either locally or on your yard.

INSURANCE

If your horse is involved in an accident where somebody is injured or something is damaged you may be found liable, so third party insurance is recommended to protect you against this potentially expensive outcome.

There are many different levels of insurance available, from basic third party, to veterinary cover for individual conditions, to the more expensive option which is lifetime cover, usually with a maximum per condition. The premium will vary according to a number of factors: the age, breed and value of your horse as well as your region, and what your horse is used for. As with any insurance policy, premiums can be reduced by adjusting your level of excess higher, although this can have the knock-on effect that it is rarely worth claiming as the bill may be only a little greater than the excess.

When you take out your policy maybe consider how much your average vet's bill is; this will vary between areas, but call-outs and subsequent follow-on visits and treatment can add up very quickly, so be realistic.

There are many different companies now providing pet insurance, so it is worth shopping around thoroughly to get the best deal, or asking your veterinary practice if there is a company that they recommend – and be sure to READ THE SMALL PRINT!

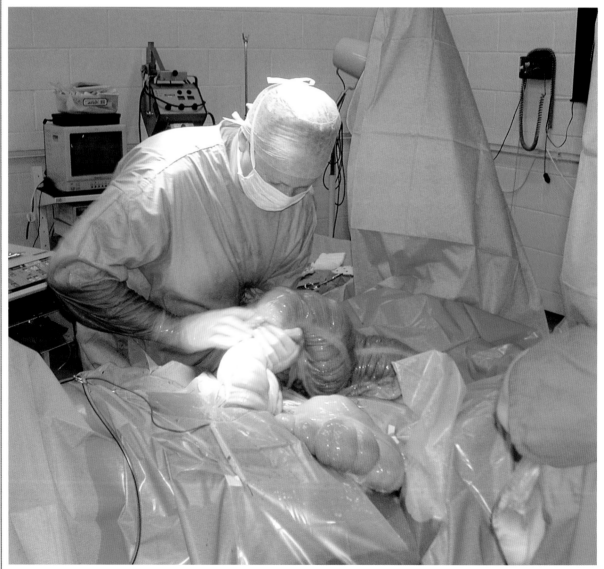

Some very advanced treatments are available but the cost can be prohibitive

GLOSSARY OF TERMS

Accessory bone Small bone at the back of the knee, very vulnerable to pressure injury under bandages.

Agonal gasps/breathing Reflex movements which look like breathing, can be made in the half an hour after death.

Anaerobic bacteria Bacteria which thrive where there is little or no oxygen, such as in a puncture wound.

Anaphylaxis An overwhelming and inappropriate immune response which can threaten life.

Antibiosis The use of antibiotics to control bacterial infection.

Axillae The equivalent of the armpit, where the front leg meets the chest.

Azoturia Muscle disorder similar to cramp, also known as exertional rhabdomyolysis.

Biochemistry Laboratory test to monitor levels of enzymes, hormones and other chemical markers in the blood.

Bog spavin Fluid build-up in the joint capsule of the hock.

Bone spavin Arthritis affecting the hock joint.

Bowed tendon Term that describes the obvious swelling of a severely strained tendon, because of the bow-like shape it makes.

Broncho-alveolar lavage Tube passed into the lower airways, guided by an endoscope until it reaches the narrowest part; sterile saline is then flushed in and sucked back to take samples of the cells and any bacterial or fungal contamination of the bronchi or alveoli.

Bursa A fluid-filled sack, similar to a joint capsule or tendon sheath, which protects a bony part of the body, such as over the withers or poll.

Cast Term to describe a horse that is lying down and unable to stand up due to lack of room, usually because it has been rolling and its legs have come up against a wall or other obstacle.

Carpus Clinical term for the knee.

Caustic cream Usually containing copper sulphate, it is used to remove proud flesh by burning away the unwanted tissue.

Cellulitis An extreme reaction normally to localized infection in the leg: the surrounding tissue swells significantly causing pain and sometimes damage to the skin.

Cirrhosis Usually affects the liver: damage from disease or toxins causes the organ to scar and shrink, and this affects the ability of the still healthy parts to function.

Colostrum The special milk made by the mare during the first day of the foal's life; it contains very high levels of antibodies that the foal's gut can only absorb during the first 12–24 hours of its life. If the foal does not receive colostrum its immune system will be seriously weakened and it is likely to require a transfusion of hyperimmune plasma to enable it to survive.

Culture Laboratory test: a swab is taken from an infected area and grown under special conditions to identify the bacteria involved.

Cushings disease A condition often seen in older horses where a benign tumour grows in the pituitary gland in the brain causing the horse to produce abnormal levels of steroids.

Cushings syndrome A term describing the collection of symptoms caused by Cushings disease. Symptoms include an increased thirst, very long haircoat regardless of season, loss of muscle mass and an increased appetite. Many horses also become prone to laminitis.

Cytology Microscopic examination of slides to determine cell type, such as inflammatory cells, bacteria, fungi, cancer cells.

Cytotoxic cream Cream used to treat sarcoids: it works by killing the cells it comes into contact with. It is only available on prescription, and must be applied by the vet.

Dermatophytosis A fungal skin infection also known as ringworm; it causes circular itchy areas on most animals and humans.

Ectoparasite Parasite that lives on the outside of the body, such as lice.

Endoparasite Parasite that lives inside the body, such as round or tape worms.

Endoscope A fibreoptic camera, usually between 1m and 1.5m long, which gives a clear picture of internal structures such as the oesophagus, airways and urinary tract.

Endocrinology Study of the hormones in the body, including reproductive hormones.

Epiglottis A structure made out of cartilage that protects the airways during swallowing; in the horse the tip usually rests on the soft palate, but it can become trapped out of position during high levels of exercise.

Epistaxis Clinical term for a nosebleed.

Equine recurrent uveitis Also known as moon blindness: an inflammation of the iris causing scarring, which affects the ability of the pupil to adjust to light.

Exertional rhabdomyolysis Muscle disorder similar to severe cramp.

Fistulous withers An infection of the bursa (fluid-filled sac) protecting the bony prominences of the spine at the withers.

Foreign body Any object found in the tissues of the body which is not part of the body, such as a splinter of wood in the skin.

Gingivitis Infection and/or inflammation of the gums; if untreated it can lead to gum recession and eventually loss of a tooth.

Granulation tissue The first stage of healing: it is very soft and bleeds easily, but has a very strong immune defence. In large wounds this is the protective layer, and skin will gradually develop on top. In some cases it can grow excessively, when it is called proud flesh.

Gutteral pouch An out-pouching of the auditory (hearing) system situated at the base of the skull.

Haematology Laboratory tests to look at the make-up of the blood, namely the number of red and white blood cells.

Haemorrhage Clinical term for bleeding.

Hausman's gag A device with spring-loaded teeth plates attached to a headcollar which allows the mouth to be opened fully and examined safely; it also allows precise dental treatment.

Histology The examination of tissues under the microscope by specialists to determine the nature of the tissue; usually used to investigate lumps that have been removed in order to diagnose whether they are cancerous or aggressive. The results can be used to guide further treatment.

151

Hydrophilic (As in dressing or gel.) Absorbent material that draws in excessive fluid such as oozing from a wound to prevent the site becoming too wet, but without allowing drying either.

Hyperimmune plasma Special intravenous treatment made from whole blood, used to treat foals that have not received adequate colostrum.

Immunosuppressed Term to describe the situation where the immune system is not working well, sometimes the case in elderly horses and young foals, and in very sick horses.

Infarction An area of dead or damaged tissue caused by loss of the blood supply, for instance because of a clot.

Joint capsule Fibrous sack surrounding the moving parts of a joint containing fluid to cushion the bones from each other.

Laminae The tissue that holds the pedal bone in position within the hoof.

Laminitis Inflammation of the tissue holding the pedal bone in position, causing severe lameness.

Lymph nodes Local centres of immunity: small glandular structures most commonly felt in the throat. An increase in their size is commonly seen in the face of infection.

Mandibular symphysis The point of the chin where the two lower jawbones meet and are fused together.

Melanoma A form of tumour seen primarily in grey horses, most often found around the anus and under the dock, but can occur anywhere in the body.

Meconium Term to describe the first faeces the foal passes: this should happen within hours of birth.

Moon blindness Also known as 'equine recurrent uveitis': a repeated inflammation of the iris causing scarring, which affects the ability of the pupil to adjust to light.

Mud fever Superficial bacterial or yeast infection of the skin, usually around the pastern and fetlock.

Navicular bone Small, crescent-shaped bone found in the foot behind the pedal bone.

Open fracture Where at least one part of a broken bone is sticking through the skin.

Osteochondritis desicans (OCD) A disorder of cartilage growth, so it weakens and flakes away from the underlying bone, causing pain, restricting joint movement, and eventually resulting in arthritis.

Pedal bone The triangular-shaped bone found in the hoof.

Pedunculated lipoma A benign fatty lump; in the abdomen these can grow on the end of a stalk, a combination that can trap and strangle portions of gut causing colic that requires surgery. This is a common cause of colic in older horses.

Pelvic flexure A narrowing of the hind gut as it does a U-turn in the pelvis; many impactions develop here, causing colic.

Peritoneum The lining round the inside of the abdomen between the organs and the muscle layer.

Poll evil Infection of the bursa protecting the bones of the spine at the poll.

Prophylactic antibiotics Antibiotic treatment used to prevent the development of infection, rather than being used to treat a current infection. For example, prior to surgery prophylactic antibiotics are used to minimize post-operative infections that will delay healing.

Proud flesh Overgrowth of the tissue of the primary stage of healing, usually when the edges of the skin do not meet.

Quidding Dropping half-chewed food due to a problem with chewing or swallowing.

Respiration Clinical term for breathing.

Sarcoid Form of skin tumour thought to be caused by a virus; it comes in many different forms, and is usually only a problem if it develops in an area where it is knocked frequently, for example under the tack.

Seedy toe Poor hoof wall structure at the toe causes splitting and weakness, and can predispose to abscess formation as the splits make it easier for infection to migrate into the hoof

Sensitivity tests (culture and sensitivity) Tests to find out which antibiotic is most effective at treating the bacteria causing disease in your horse.

Septic arthritis Bacterial infection in the joint capsule.

Septicaemia A very serious infection where the bacteria has reached the bloodstream.

Sequestrum Fragment of bone without a blood supply which produces a foreign body reaction.

Serum Fluid part of the blood once the red and white blood cells have been removed.

Shockwave therapy The use of ultrasonic waves to stimulate blood flow and speed up healing while reducing the build-up of scar tissue.

Splint Term used to describe the bony thickening which results from a fracture or sprain of the splint bone.

Splint bone The remnant of the metacarpal bones. Horses are mammals so originally had five metacarpals, the equivalent of those in the human hand.

Stem cell therapy The use of cells harvested from the sternum of a horse, cultured in a special laboratory, and then injected into damaged tendon to promote healing without the formation of scar tissue. Still in the very early stages of research, this treatment is only available at referral centres.

Tendon sheath A tough protective layer covering the tendon, within which it can stretch or contract smoothly.

Tetanus A bacterial infection (*Clostridium tetani*) that produces a toxin causing all the muscles in the body to become stiff and inflexible; it is usually caused by soil contamination of an open wound, and can be fatal if not recognized and treated early.

Thrush Yeast or fungal infection of the heel or sole of the foot caused by being permanently wet.

Tracheal wash Diagnostic technique performed in conjunction with endoscopy. A volume of sterile saline is introduced into the airways just before the trachea divides into bronchi, and is then collected for cytology and culture.

Tushes Residual canine teeth, most commonly seen in male horses.

Uveitis Inflammation of the iris, a recurrent condition in horses, also known as moon blindness. The inflamed iris prevents the pupil from contracting and dilating in a normal manner.

Vasodilator A drug which dilates the blood vessels.

Viraemia A chronic condition where a virus becomes resident in the body, usually causing chronic debilitation and general poor health, without specific symptoms.

INDEX

153